YOUR LIFE
TRAIN FOR IT

Bear Grylls

with Natalie Summers

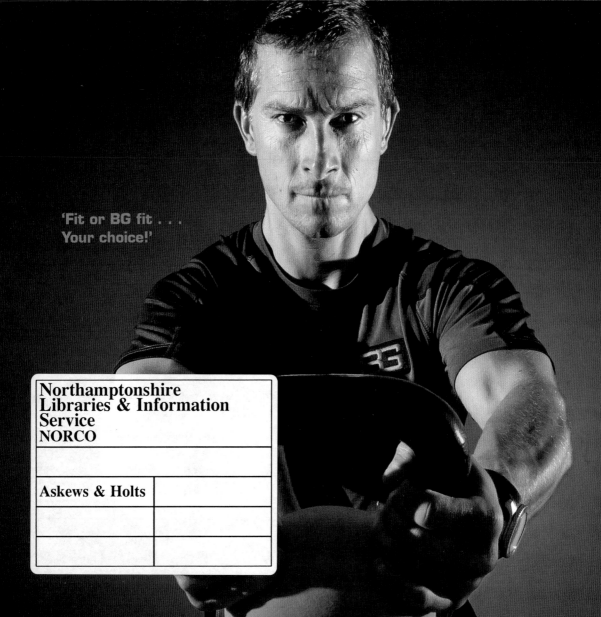

'Fit or BG fit . . .
Your choice!'

I would like to dedicate this book to Natalie and the BG EPIC Training team,
who have worked so hard to bring this style of Express High Intensity Interval
Training to everyday people looking to get fitter, leaner and stronger
than they ever imagined possible.

This is right at the heart of what we stand for and together there are few
missions as fun as building a community of like-minded enthusiasts and
helping people achieve their fitness goals.

Natalie, you have done so much for me in guiding us down this road of
endeavour and positive change – and you have made it all so much fun!

Here's to the continued adventure . . .

CONTENTS

INTRODUCTION

**First up, I am not a natural athlete.
And boy I wish I was!**

All my life, from school, through the military
and then into the climbing and expedition
fraternity, I so often found myself surrounded
by people who effortlessly accomplished feats
of dizzying strength, endurance and agility.
And to top it all, they hardly ever seemed to
train. I was always sick with envy.

But the truth is, very few of us are made
like that. For most of the world – me included
– getting and staying fit, building real muscle
power, flexibility and stamina, takes time, hard
work and dedication.

It also takes knowledge, and that is where
this book comes in.

I spent years of my life trying and trying
to get lean and ripped – but I was busy going
about it in all the wrong ways. I would train
and train but I would never change very much.
What I did have, though, was the fire and
determination to persevere, to adapt, to train
even harder – and somehow to try to close
the gulf between me and those many natural
athletes who inhabited my world.

And it kind of worked. I got fit, and strong,
and bendy. I persevered where many would
have fallen by the wayside. I achieved those
summits and those military badges. But
looking at me, you'd never have believed it, as I
never really looked that strong or fit. And, if I'm
really honest, I wanted to. I know it's a bit vain
to say it, but I didn't just want to *be* fit and
strong; I wanted to *look* it too.

So I bought the books. But what is it with
most fitness books?! Where we seek inspiration
we often find intimidation, and where we hope
to discover a way to look and feel fitter we
often experience a sense of 'How can I ever
measure up to that?' But I read them anyway.
And I kept training. I had a goal.

One other thing that motivated me was
that I didn't want to get old and look back and
think, wow, I never managed to walk on my
hands, or I never could swing my body round
a pull-up bar, or do back somersaults, or back
flips, or touch my head on my knees. So I learnt
how to do all that. I almost killed myself a few
times in the process, but I stuck at it and I did
it. The hard way.

But I still looked the same, and I couldn't
quite understand it. Then doubt crept in. And
so I convinced myself that maybe we are a
product of our genes and that we can't really
change how we look, feel or perform to any
great extent. I began to believe that I could
never *look* really fit as well as *be* really fit.

Yet still part of me was determined to make
changes happen – to find a smarter and more
effective way to achieve my fitness aims of
functional strength, endurance and flexibility;
to make me lean, fast and ripped. That was the
goal.

My military training and then my
mountaineering had helped me build up decent
endurance and strength, but when I started
filming survival shows I really began to require
lean strength, speed and flexibility – not just
brute power.

So I got busy. Motivated by a partially
flawed mix of pride, vanity and the fact that
my job was demanding a certain type of
fitness, I started on a quest to try all the fitness

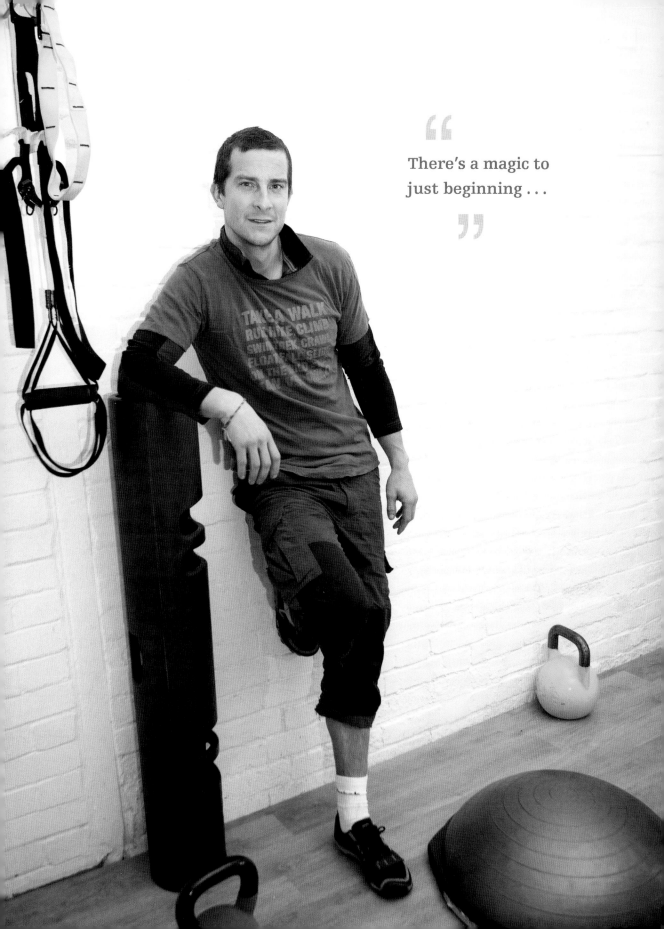

"
There's a magic to
just beginning . . .

"

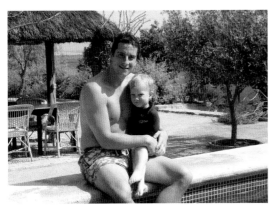

Post military and Everest I definitely let it go for a few years. Aged twenty-nine, I was a stone and a half heavier than I am now.

programmes out there. And I did them all. Well, at least a ton of them. I fell flat on my face a few times – sometimes literally – but slowly I began to learn what worked and what didn't.

I was searching for a style of training that was fast, efficient and achievable. I wanted a regime that was also fun, dynamic and – above all – gave real results to regular folk.

It wasn't an easy thing to find.

Then, through a friend, and a load of recommendations, I started training regularly with Natalie, one on one – and very soon it kind of felt like the scales were falling from my eyes.

I was training in a way that I never had before. The workouts were not only much shorter than I had ever been used to, they were also much harder! They weren't based around lifting heavy weights for endless sets, nor did they involve miles and miles of running, or boring, repetitive routines.

Instead, the training was always functional and core-based – meaning that it never targeted muscles in isolation. Instead, every exercise I did worked on multiple parts of the body and they were exercises I had never even come across before. It was never just a push-up, but instead it would be a push-up on one foot with the other knee up by my elbow. Sometimes done explosively or sometimes done as slow isometric exercises. The workouts were always done to a clock – intense movements followed by a brief few seconds of rest, then back in.

This was a programme that seemed to combine the best of cardio, weight training, yoga and the increasingly popular HIIT – High Intensity Interval Training – all in one.

The workouts were based on three training disciplines: Kettlebell Resistance training, Bodyweight training and flexibility/Primal Power Stretch training (all of which are explained in more depth in Section 2).

Soon I noticed almost every newspaper and fitness magazine was beginning to recognize the results that can come from this type of cross-training. And of course by now Natalie and I had been doing it for over two years. I loved that we seemed to be ahead of the curve!

Above all, I found my body shape was starting to change. All the time, I was getting trimmer, fitter and more flexible. I was getting faster, more dynamic and stronger. And what was so crazy was that it wasn't taking me six hours a day (like I kept hearing that Madonna was doing!). Here I was, training hard and intensively for just a maximum of 30 minutes. I felt almost guilty! How could this be working?

We would sometimes shorten the workouts even more, doing ultra high-intensity workouts of just 10 minutes – but normally we would never train any longer than 30 minutes. This in itself was a game-changer for me. Could I really get substantial, tangible benefits and results in so short a time? Could I really get lean, ripped, flexible, strong and fast in under 30 minutes, a few days a week?

My body seemed to think so, and I noticed that invariably my muscles were still twitching some four hours later in a way I had never experienced through conventional programmes.

That after-burn (see page 10) was a good thing – it signalled that there had been shock to the muscles, which meant stimulation and growth, plus it meant I would be calorie-burning as well, long after the session had finished.

I knew neither of those things happen when you just run or do repetitive weights.

So I kept training. Kept changing.

I also began to see more and more research supporting this view that short, sharp, intense training has a much more beneficial and lasting fat-burning effect than long, slow runs or gym sessions. I read about the dramatic health benefits to cholesterol and much more. But, above all, I loved the fact that as I was getting older, I was getting fitter than ever before.

I also made the effort to educate myself in the other part of the equation: good nutrition. This is something they definitely never taught in school, or in the military. Yet it is one of the most critical building blocks for achieving optimum fitness. So I read and studied, and I learnt. I re-trained myself to experiment and discover the delicious tastes of real, whole foods, as found in nature. I learnt how most of us have been brought up with an all-too-common addiction to salt, sugar and fat, all of which detract from the incredible taste and nutrient absorption of whole, natural, life-enhancing foods.

I am certain you will love the part of this book that touches on nutrition. It has been an eye-opener for me, and in the most positive of ways – for lean, good health and longevity.

Anyway, here I am at thirty-nine, and I am fitter, leaner, faster and more flexible than at any other time before. It has been an incredible journey, and I only wish I had learnt all this earlier.

I now train no more than four or five days a week for 30 minutes at a time. I eat better, more delicious food than in the past, and I look and feel the way I wished I did when I was twenty-one (and surrounded by all those natural athletes I was talking about!).

In short, my life has changed dramatically because of this revolutionary style of training.

This book is all about how you can do it too.

Are you ready for the journey?

It's your life. Train for it.

OK, let's go do it.

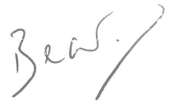

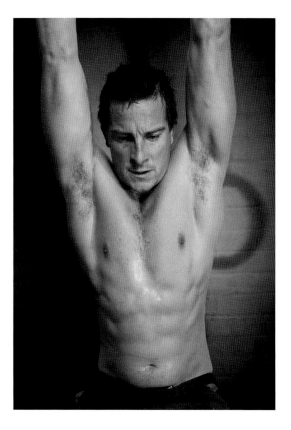

The leaner, fitter, healthier me (aged thirty-nine)!

1 | TRAINING PRINCIPLES

The training principles you are about to read have empowered me physically and mentally, and have massively enriched my life. If you adopt the same or similar principles, I know they will do the same for you.

There are four key principles underlying all my training:

- train with purpose
- train hard and short
- make it progressive and diverse
- focus on functional and core training

Let's go through these one by one, as good foundations are so important when you train. Solid principles sustain you through the hard times and give you a vision beyond the pain.

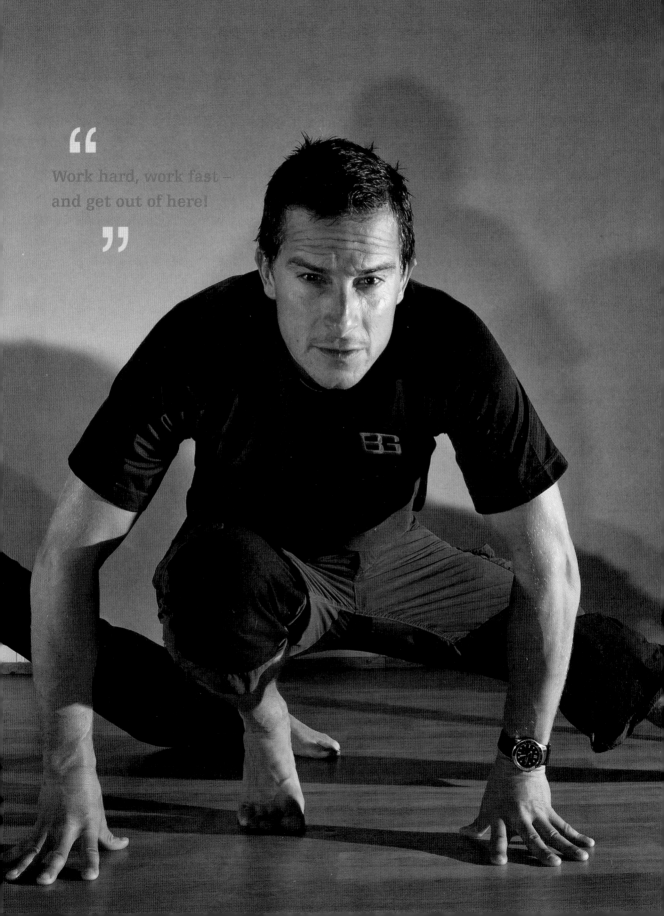

"
Work hard, work fast –
and get out of here!

"

TRAIN WITH PURPOSE

'This training is building you into a strong, flexible, lean, powerful, dynamic athlete.'

One of my key principles is to train with purpose and intent, towards a clear, tangible, achievable goal. This is the goal or the purpose of this style of training:

- a high level of cardiovascular fitness – *a strong and healthy heart*
- a high level of muscular fitness – *endurance and strength*
- a good range of motion in your joints – *flexibility*
- improved motor skills (i.e. the ability of your brain and nervous system to control your body's movement) – *agility, speed, balance, coordination, power and swift reaction times*
- a knowledgeable and well-balanced approach to nutrition and your daily diet
- reaching your target weight/lean muscle mass
- the ability to cope with the stresses and strains of your daily life and sustain social relationships

TRAIN HARD AND SHORT

'It's all about intensity, not duration.'

Yep, another of my principles is to train hard for a short period of time. We call this 'express training'. Why do I train like this? Because, in a nutshell, it works and who doesn't want more results in less time?!

These short bursts of training are designed to fit in with our busy schedules, whether it's 30 minutes before work, or in your lunch break, all the way down to grabbing 3 minutes whilst travelling or between meetings.

So, the express workouts in this book last between 3 and 30 minutes, but no longer. Since starting this type of training, I've increased my overall fitness, developed leaner muscle mass, increased my strength and flexibility – all as a result of these short-interval, high-intensity workouts. I no longer train relentlessly for hours on end and am in much better shape than before because of it.

If you're like me, you might find it hard to recondition yourself to train for short times like this, but trust me on this one – if you follow these programmes and stick to the shorter, more intense time periods, then the results will be dramatic.

The express workouts are all about metabolic conditioning and using structured interval training. That means we use active and rest intervals that maximize the efficiency of your body's energy system.

OK, so what does this actually mean? Well, the high-interval, high-intensity approach to exercise results in a response known as the 'after-burn' effect, which translates to an increase in metabolic function following vigorous or strenuous exercise. Simply put, your body will carry on using energy after you have finished your workout. This occurs because it takes more energy and time for your body to recover after high-intensity workouts than after steady-paced workouts.

Here is where your commitment comes in! To get the maximum results and the desired response from your body you will need to do the following in *every* workout:

Get sweaty, really sweaty!
Not sweating is not a sign of fitness, so don't hold back. You have to go for it. But remember, it's not for long – you can do anything for 20 or 30 seconds. And in 30 minutes max you will be done and feeling amazing! So learn to love sweating!

To get sweaty you need to work hard.
To work hard you need to be working close to, or at, maximum effort. Working out at maximum effort means you will be breathing heavily. This type of training is just as cardio-based as it is strength- and speed-based. If you can hold a steady conversation during your workout, you are not working hard enough and you are limiting the after-burn effect. Commit to the short work periods, train hard and your body will respond.

Experience the burn.
Regardless of the type of discipline you are using (Kettlebell, Bodyweight or Primal Power Stretch), you are aiming to find the point where you feel you cannot complete another repetition or movement – we call it the burn. To reach your point of failure in the work periods, add intensity by lifting a heavier kettlebell, work faster on bodyweight exercises, or find greater depth in your stretching poses.

By applying these express training methods and working out at high intensities you are asking your heart and lungs to work extra hard, so as well as reaping the benefits of that after-burn effect, you will be massively improving your cardiovascular capacity too!

I know this from experience, as after I started training like this I stopped running. Then, six months later, I went for a run with a friend on a route we both knew well, and I was noticeably faster and less out of breath than I had ever been before on this trail. This was due to the simple fact that my new high-intensity functional training had given me a much better cardiovascular fitness than I had ever got just by running steadily and regularly. This surprised me at the time but now I understand the principles of why.

So learn to embrace the burn and fatigue in short bursts.

To recap the benefits, you will:

- Increase your fitness and cardiovascular efficiency – the high-intensity intervals increase your body's ability to deliver oxygen to your working muscles. You work your body hard and it responds to the physical challenge, so making you fitter.
- Burn more body fat and maintain lean muscle – your body uses up energy from your fat stores.
- Experience a rise in your metabolism – the 'after-burn' effect.

It didn't take me long to get used to working at a high intensity, but it did take a while to get to grips with letting go during the scheduled rests. You can't go flat out all the time – it is the combination of intense work then rest that forms a substantial part of our training style.

These work-rest intervals optimize your body's ability to burn fat and help determine the way energy is made available to your muscles.

By not holding back during the rest interval, you risk turning your exercising into an aerobic workout, reducing the efficiency of your body to burn fat.

The workouts in this book make equal use of both active and rest intervals. I endeavour always to train hard right to the last millisecond in the work period *but* only safely in the knowledge that the short rest time is just one breath away!

The workouts in this book are based on the following training methods:

High Intensity Interval Training (HIIT)

Exercise blocks that involve working at maximum intensity for short periods of time separated with a rest or low-intensity interval.

Tabata

A form of HIIT, tabata is a 4-minute exercise block. It requires you to work at maximum effort for 20 seconds followed by a complete rest interval of 10 seconds for 8 rounds.

Density

A minimum of 3 minutes of continuous effort followed by a rest period. Typically, the intensity level is medium to high due to the length of the active intervals.

As many rounds as possible (AMRAP)

This involves completing a circuit of exercises as one round and then completing as many more rounds of that circuit as possible within a set time. The hardest part of this training method is remembering how many rounds you have completed, although counting can also be a welcome distraction from the pain! AMRAP, though, is a great method for tracking and testing your fitness and for measuring your fitness gains on your journey to total physical fitness. (See Tracking Your Progress, page 198.)

PROGRESSION + DIVERSITY = INEVITABLE CHANGE

Your body is going to change for the better! The reasons for the positive changes I've experienced are down to the **diversity** of the exercises I undertake and the **progression** of my training.

We all have favourite exercises that we absolutely love and have mastered, but if we continue to do them with no progression we won't challenge our bodies and the results won't come. This is the cycle I was in for many years. Doing the same runs or same circuits over and over again. Isn't that the definition of madness? Doing the same thing over and over and expecting different results?!

Yes, it's good to master the exercise, but then you have to make sure to evolve it and make it more challenging so that you progress.

You don't have to be an expert to think of how to progress an exercise. Take basic push-ups as an example. Once you can do them with relative ease, you can progress them by starting to raise one of your legs off the floor, or progressing to a single-hand push-up. Listen to your body: if it is working harder then you have progressed the move.

Here are some ideas to consider when designing your workout to ensure progression:

- If you are using kettlebells, gradually increase the weight of your kettlebell.
- Vary the intensity of a workout: push yourself to work harder.
- Increase the duration of workouts – for example, from 10 minutes to a maximum of 30 minutes.
- Increase the number of repetitions of the exercises within each interval.

Use your progression charts and fitness evaluations (see pages 203–6) to track how your fitness changes.

FUNCTIONAL AND CORE TRAINING

My entire training ethos is based around 'functional' training. Functional training is about having the physical strength, core stability and freedom of movement to be able to do things that beforehand you would never have believed possible, or that maybe you had lost through age or neglect. I have too many friends who have big biceps but bad backs; or big quads but they can't touch their toes. They have no all-round dynamic fitness and they suffer as a result.

Functional fitness is about having the body nature intended you to have in order to survive. Our ancestors needed to be fast and therefore lean; strong in short bursts; and flexible enough to reach, climb and fight – all in order to avoid getting eaten by a wild animal or attacked by marauding neighbours!

Our bodies want to be strong, flexible, fast, lean and dynamic – this is how we are meant to be. We aren't designed to be beefcakes!

Put simply, functional training will prepare you for life!

All the workouts in this book have been designed to focus on this functional and core training. This in turn improves overall muscular strength and endurance, cardiovascular performance, flexibility and motor/skills fitness, as well as 'core stability'.

Core stability is the effective use of the trunk muscles and the shoulder girdle to support the spine and allow your limbs to move freely. Adding core training to your workouts will help improve posture and reduce injury. It also enhances agility and leads to improved balance and coordination as well as increased power and speed – all of which are critical in my job.

By the way, this core focus is why the people I know who have the best abs are so often also the ones who hardly do any regular sit-ups. Instead, their whole workouts are so core-focused that their deep abs are being effectively exercised all the time, almost without them knowing it.

Here is one of my favourite tabata blocks for core training:

CORE TABATA
Time: 4 minutes
Mixed discipline

Complete the following sequence of exercises. Work for 20 seconds and rest for 10 seconds between exercises.

- Turkish Get-up Half, right (see page 57)
- Turkish Get-up Half, left
- Kettlebell Single-arm Plank, right (see page 41)
- Kettlebell Single-arm Plank, left
- High Plank Superman, on your hands and feet (see page 97)
- Spider Side Plank, right (see page 64)
- Spider Side Plank, left
- High Plank Superman, on your hands and feet

OK, so those are the principles on which I base my training. Those are the foundations upon which we can now go and build the workouts. We know our purpose and goals, we train hard and short. We make sure the workouts are always progressive and changing, and we keep the focus on functional and core training in everything we do.

It's time now to look at the three different training disciplines we are going to use . . .

2 | TRAINING DISCIPLINES:

KETTLEBELL, BODYWEIGHT AND PRIMAL POWER STRETCH

'The will to win means nothing without the will to train.'

This section introduces the training methods that form the cornerstones of my training regime:

- Kettlebell Resistance training
- Bodyweight training
- Primal Power Stretch training

KETTLEBELL RESISTANCE TRAINING

'Kettlebells work the core muscular infrastructure like no machine or barbell ever can!'

Anatomy of a kettlebell

What is a kettlebell? Quite simply, it's a cast-iron, ball-shaped weight with a single handle and can vary in weight from 2kg to in excess of 48kg. They originated in the seventeenth century when, although originally used as a tool for weighing grain, during relaxation periods in the working day men started to use them in competitions of strength.

Over time the appeal of the kettlebell has continued to grow. Its most recent popularity has been spurred on by the many benefits associated with the discipline, in particular how Kettlebell Resistance training promotes core training by using basic human movement patterns – hence they are a key component to effective functional training (see Functional and Core Training, page 13).

Unlike other traditional resistance equipment, like barbells or dumbells, the weight of a kettlebell is not evenly distributed because of its unique shape.

This creates a natural imbalance as you use it, which helps activate your stabilization muscles (the muscles that support your trunk), making kettlebells an incredibly effective training tool to increase and improve your core strength.

Why train with a kettlebell?

Natalie and I both love training with kettlebells. They are the ultimate, versatile workout tool for challenging, varied and effective training. Here is why.

Kettlebells are a form of resistance training – a discipline that concentrates on working with weights to build strength and muscle mass, improve bone density and raise metabolism.

We implemented Kettlebell Resistance training into my regular workouts as a full-body conditioning programme to improve my power generation, muscular strength, core strength, and also to help strengthen the muscles in my back. (You might remember I once broke my back in three places during a freefall parachuting accident whilst I was serving with 21 SAS. Doctors told me that I would be unable to return to active duty as I would never recover the strength in my back to carry the backpack, weaponry and supplies that I was able to cross mountains and jungles with before. I like to think this training has helped me prove them wrong!)

Other benefits of training with kettlebells include:

- improved cardiovascular fitness
- reduced body fat and increased lean muscle
- improved bone health
- enhanced coordination
- increased core strength
- improved range of movement and joint mobility
- greater joint and ligament strength
- a quick, effective and fun workout!

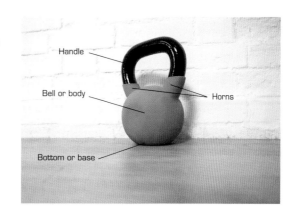

By adding a Kettlebell Resistance workout into your training twice a week you will really start to experience all the benefits above.

During the workouts we will guide you on correct kettlebell form, in particular which grip position you should use (see Kettlebell Grips, pages 28–9).

BODYWEIGHT TRAINING

I love Bodyweight training and I continue to be amazed by just how difficult it can be to lift your own weight when you start messing with your body and putting it in strange positions! Using your body as resistance is a super-efficient, versatile and, above all, convenient way to work out, especially if you have a busy work and home life, as so many of us do.

All you need is your body, your commitment and a little imagination. Throw in our express timing and principles, and the fitness gains will soon become apparent. As always, you have to work hard in the active intervals, rest adequately in between and fuel your body properly at the end (see Fuel and Recovery, page 190)! Remember, exercise mimics life: you get out what you put in!

Here are just a few of the changes that I have noticed since adding a Bodyweight discipline to my workouts:

TRAINING DISCIPLINES

Improved athletic performance.

I've built speed and improved my explosive power: I can jump further, higher, faster and can keep jumping for longer than ever before. (Note to self: useful in the mountains and jungles!)

Reduced body fat.

Bodyweight training has dramatically raised my metabolic rate, which in turn keeps my body burning calories like a furnace for hours after I have stopped training (see 'after-burn' effect, page 10). My percentage of body fat has gone down dramatically as a result of this style of training.

Enhanced flexibility.

Not only has my muscle strength and endurance improved, but the bodyweight combinations and circuits I use have enhanced my suppleness, flexibility and core strength. As the bulk of the exercises involve a real dependence on my core to execute the moves with correct technique, I've seen a massive improvement in my ability to hold even the most complex of plank positions. Something I probably couldn't do even at the height of my military fitness aged twenty-one. Even though I was able to carry huge weights across the mountains for long periods of time, my functional bodyweight strength was poor.

Increased cardiovascular fitness.

By employing the training methods described in the box on page 12 and combining a number of exercises together (such as a Burpee and Primal Push-up combination), my cardiovascular capacity has improved no end. It's amazing how just working out with pure bodyweight moves gets my heart pumping like I am sprinting on a very steep hill run!

Enjoyment!

I'm finally enjoying training and working out in a way I have rarely done before. When I'm travelling or pushed for time, I play around with numerous combinations of exercises in the Bodyweight discipline. When you've got to grips with the moves, start experimenting with this: have a look at how to build a unique Bodyweight workout for yourself (see page 186). Here is one that the crew and I used recently whilst waiting on a jungle airstrip in Panama – go on, give it a go!

- 8 Pull-ups, wide grip (see page 90)
- 8 Single-leg Push-ups, right (see page 94)
- 8 Single-leg Push-ups, left
- 6 Pull-ups, wide grip
- 6 Single-leg Push-ups, right
- 6 Single-leg Push-ups, left
- 4 Pull-ups, wide grip
- 4 Single-leg Push-ups, right
- 4 Single-leg Push-ups, left
- 2 Pull-ups, wide grip
- 2 Single-leg Push-ups, right
- 2 Single-leg Push-ups, left
- 30 seconds High Knees, with arms (see page 76)
- 30 seconds Cross Mountain Climbers with Push-up (see page 66)
- 30 seconds High to Low Planks (see page 62)

Rest for 2 minutes.
Repeat if you dare!

PRIMAL POWER STRETCH TRAINING

'Unclutter your mind, be stronger, stand taller and move freely.'

These yoga-inspired power workouts allow me to incorporate a flexibility discipline into my training regime that is critical for me in so many ways.

After my parachuting accident, I spent almost a year in and out of military rehabilitation centres. I went through very intense treatment including physiotherapy, hydrotherapy, osteotherapy and everything in between. Still my back hurt like hell. A year or so on, I discovered that I needed a good strong sports physio-massage once a week to manage the pain, keep me straight and free up the muscles and scar tissue. Otherwise I would start to really suffer.

Eventually, almost out of desperation, I took up yoga. It felt amazing. The poses lengthened and strengthened my back muscles, broke down the scar tissue and straightened me out, mentally as well as physically! On top of this, I found that I no longer needed the massages. I was hooked! Since then I've worked with Natalie to adapt those poses into very functional power stretch workouts that give me all the benefits of yoga, coupled to strengthening exercises within the poses. We call it Primal Power and it kicks ass!

As a result, I have a greater range of movement than ever before, my back no longer hurts like it used to, and I am much less prone to injury than so many people who train a lot. And if I do ever fall over or down something – which happens quite a lot when filming out in the wild – I've noticed that I'm so much more bendy and able to absorb the impact than before. (In fact, looking back, I reckon the bendy joints and flexible muscles I've

developed through Primal Power have saved me a bunch of times!)

Primal Power also allows me to enjoy that sense of calm that comes with the massive endorphin release just after primal training! It's like nice Bear has come back into town! (Ask Shara!)

In short, Primal Power fuses all the best elements from traditional yoga, Pilates, flexibility and strength training into one challenging express workout using active and static strength. Combined with our express training methods, it creates a dynamic and effective workout that will keep your body moving freely in the way it was designed to do.

Like me, you will find that Primal Power Stretch:

- increases flexibility
- improves posture and spinal alignment
- improves muscular strength and stamina
- improves balance and coordination
- activates your core

Primal Power has also allowed me to take all sorts of leaps of faith in life, both mentally and physically. The workouts help me feel grounded and centred in a way that is hard to explain. Maybe it's the very contact of bare feet and balance exercises on hard floor, or the 'head time' in which I get to pray for the things that matter most to me. Either way, at the end of training I always feel better equipped to tackle the daily battles that we all have to deal with in life.

Challenges are inevitable, but defeat is optional!

Primal Power Stretch workouts sit perfectly within a functional fitness-training regime as they help to develop a strong, supple body, alert mind and injury-free existence (see Functional and Core Training, page 13).

3 | GET READY TO TRAIN

So you're about to begin this journey to a fitter, leaner, stronger, more flexible you. But before we begin, there are a few final but important points to put into your brain. It will take a second to read but could make a critical difference in the long run. So here goes . . .

EXERCISE SAFELY

OK, I'm going to take you through some quick health-and-safety screening. I think people often like to think that I am a danger junkie who eats risk for breakfast, but actually the truth is that I am still alive because I have learnt when to be smart and cautious and when to be bold. It is a key skill: play the right card at the right time. And experience has taught me that all too often it is ego that gets people killed. So here we are: stay alive, be smart!

'Yep, I'm fit enough to train!'

Are you? Now you don't have to be an elite athlete to follow my workouts, but if you have any pre-existing medical conditions or an injury that could be exacerbated by participating in physical activity, please seek medical clearance before you begin.

When Bear first arrived at my studio, like all clients I requested him to complete a Physical Activity Readiness Questionnaire (PARQ), which is a simple evaluation to make sure you are physically able to exercise. Bear filled it in and stated that he had no pre-existing medical conditions and no pre-existing injuries that might affect physical activity. Awesome! A model client!

However, imagine my shock when months later I read his Wikipedia entry:

'In 1996, Bear suffered a free-fall parachuting accident in Zambia. His canopy ripped at 4,900 metres (16,000 ft), partially opening, causing Bear to fall and land on his parachute pack on his back, which partially crushed three vertebrae.'

Panic hit me, but by this time it was too late. I'd already started Bear on a training programme and I couldn't really turn him away at this stage – especially now that the workouts were starting to yield such great results for him!

But with Bear's history now highlighted, I began to incorporate a back-strengthening and conditioning element to our workouts.

This may make you smile, but when it comes to exercise it is important for your own personal safety that you are honest in terms of your abilities, limitations and injury history. We all know we can achieve anything we put our minds to, but when participating in exercise it is critical to start and continue safely. With this in mind, I have designed a simple PARQ to provide guidance if you are unsure of your readiness to exercise (see page 198).

Use the correct technique at the correct level!

The workouts in this book use express training methods, which will raise your heart rate and make you sweat. This is a good thing! Performed correctly, the workouts are safe and effective, but take care to check your technique. If you have not exercised for a prolonged period of time, adapt your training to suit your level.

To do this we advise you to:

- Start at a lower effort level, for example 60–70% of your maximum effort within the interval, and build up to the recommended effort level of 75–85%. A good way of measuring your percentage of effort is to think of it as a scale of 1–10, with 1 equalling 10% effort and 10 equalling 100% effort.

- Opt for a lighter weight for Kettlebell training (see page 20).

- Choose a shorter-duration exercise block.

As your fitness and confidence progress, gradually increase the intensity, weight and duration of your workouts.

The workouts will challenge your body, so make sure you warm up and cool down properly (see pages 128–39) to maximize your training results.

Environment and equipment safety

Before you begin, complete a quick, visual risk assessment of your training environment. It might seem obvious, but ensure you do the following:

- Look for any objects or obstacles on the floor – clear them away if they are likely to get in your way.

- Make sure that the floor isn't slippery.
- Ensure that you have enough space to jump up and move sideways.
- Make sure you are wearing appropriate clothing (see below).
- Be very careful if there are other people nearby, especially children.
- If you are going to be doing kettlebell workouts, be aware that you will be swinging around a heavy, cast-iron object that could cause damage or injury if used incorrectly. Take care to learn how to hold your kettlebell correctly using the recommended grips (see pages 28–9).

WHAT YOU WILL NEED

All the training disciplines and methods have been designed to use either no equipment or minimal equipment. You don't need a fancy gym membership, specialist clothing or trendy gadgets to gain great results! The only investments we recommend you make are:

- A kettlebell (or two if your budget allows). If you are new to this form of training, we suggest an 8kg kettlebell. For intermediate kettlebell practitioners, we recommend a 12–16kg kettlebell and for experienced users a 20+kg kettlebell.

- A mat. A good exercise mat will provide a little comfort for floor work. Make sure it's at least as long as you are tall to allow you to do some of the Primal Power Stretch exercises lying down.

- Some suitable clothing. Wear clothing that is comfortable and won't detract from your workout. Bodyweight and Primal Power Stretch can be done barefoot, but wear appropriate training shoes for the Kettlebell workouts.

YOUR PROGRESS

Before you embark on your unique fitness journey, take my advice: plan it and start writing stuff down!

Seriously, think about what it is you want to achieve – it's always useful to have a starting point, whether it's accomplishing discipline-specific fitness goals (something as simple as completing a pull-up!), achieving weight loss or a reduction in body fat, or simply desiring a better lifestyle. Having such goals in mind is a great start, but when you commit them to paper your targets become tangible and real.

As my mum used to say: a goal without a date on it is just a wish!

Working out goals can sometimes be the hardest part. Generally most people want to be fitter, have better muscle definition and look like a cover model – and that's just us guys! These are great goals, but if you really want to achieve maximum fitness results you need to drive down further and set realistic, well-defined and measurable small goals as part of your ultimate, overarching fitness target.

Keeping your goals small will help you successfully reach them. The first goal might be as simple as waking up early to complete a 3-minute density exercise block every other day for ten days.

Starting any fitness regime is a commitment and the reality is that you have to make time for it. But rather than looking at it as a chore, think about each workout as being a positive step towards a fitter, leaner, stronger you. The reality is that you *can* choose to make time to exercise, particularly when you're embracing time-efficient, express training – which is exactly what these workouts are.

The key to making working out into a habit is to schedule it into your diary. Don't be afraid to move other things around to accommodate exercise. After all, regular exercise helps create a healthy body and mind, and by adopting a structured and committed exercise regime you will start to see an upswing in productivity in other areas of your life and work.

Start prioritizing ruthlessly, and if that means getting into the habit of waking up 15 minutes early to exercise, then do it! Habits and actions create success and breed motivation.

I have a simple rule for when I am feeling unmotivated and not in the mood to train. I simply commit to doing the first 3 minutes of the workout, and if I still want to quit after that, then I can. Invariably what happens is that after a few minutes the blood is flowing, my motivation picks up and I am excited to get the workout done and finished!

It sounds simple and crazy, but it helps me so often. Whatever works for you, find a 'hot button' that will keep you going and training. Remember: consistency is key if you want to see change.

Make a start by completing the short fitness evaluation test on page 202. Creating a personal progress chart is the next step and a key element in helping you achieve total physical fitness and keeping you focused. You can use the one on pages 203–6 to help. All great journeys need a starting point.

My personal progress charts are scribbled on the wall in my 'man cave', where I often train at home, along with all of the workouts you are about to experience. It makes it easy for me to mix up my training and keep it fresh. Plus, keeping track of my progress lets me know how far I have come and how far I still have to go, which is key to motivation.

HOW TO TRAIN

When it comes to achieving tangible fitness results, you have to look at the time you spend training and the intensity of your workouts.

For the best results, my rule of thumb is to train in intervals of maximum effort, or as close to maximum effort as possible, for 30 minutes a day, a minimum of 4 days a week. You should aim for 1–2 active recovery days/rest days. What this translates into is actually only about 2 hours a week! And I am way fitter on this regime than when I was training every day for an hour or more!

Less is so often more, and even by committing to a 4-minute high intensity workout on a daily basis your body will experience the 'after-burn' effect. Some research suggests completing a 4-minute workout can be more beneficial than an hour of running, with multiple health benefits way beyond just fitness.

Scheduling Rest and Active Recovery Days and Training Breaks

'Repair, rebuild, relax and strengthen.'

Active recovery and rest days are an essential part of any high-intensity workout programme. They can help reduce training stress, repair damage from high-intensity training days and reduce the effects of overtraining.

A rest day is just that: a complete rest from *any* training. However, it doesn't mean a rest from good nutrition. Don't allow any rest days you schedule to become 'cheat days'. Be sure you focus on eating well (see Fuel and Recovery, page 190) to help your body repair and rebuild itself, and get stronger.

An active recovery day consists of training at a lower intensity, approximately 60% effort. The aim of any active recovery workout is to get blood back into the muscles you have worked the previous day to maximize and improve recovery. They can also help ease any delayed-onset muscle soreness or stiffness you may experience after completing high-intensity workouts.

Active recovery days are there for those who are not exercising at 80–100% effort in every session. If you are new to exercise, aim to build in an active recovery workout a minimum of twice a week and, if you're more experienced, a minimum of once a week.

Primal Power Stretch is a great discipline for an active recovery workout by training at 60% of your maximum effort, but you could also go swimming, walking or simply complete a full-body stretch.

If you're the type of athlete who will go 'all out' in every session no matter what the discipline, then a complete rest day once a week, which will allow both your body and mind a break from training, is recommended.

Rest days can also be used if you experience any signs of overtraining:

■ prolonged feeling of muscle heaviness and soreness post-training
■ illness
■ increased injury
■ insomnia
■ depression
■ no progression in fitness level

Listen to your body and if you think you may be overtraining, schedule a rest day.

Scheduled Training Breaks
A scheduled training break is a longer period of consecutive rest and recovery days that allows your body to recover fully, recharge, progress your fitness and reduce your risk of injury. Every six weeks Bear has a scheduled training break from all high-intensity and resistance training, typically made up of:

1 active recovery day + 2 rest days + 1 active recovery day = training break

It is better to start small and build up than to go out all guns blazing and then run out of ammo after a week!

The workouts on pages 128–79 are the heart of this book and the key to how I maintain and have built my fitness. From flexibility to the ability to lift heavy kettlebells with ease, used correctly these workouts will help you achieve amazing results and will give you everything you need to get strong and stay fit for life.

I have organized the workouts into different sections for ease of use:

■ You can choose to follow the Focused Workouts in Kettlebell, Bodyweight or Primal Power Stretch disciplines (see pages 142–65) for a structured and guided approach to your training.
■ For a real challenge, check out the Hero workouts on pages 166–79.
■ Alternatively, for a more personalized approach, you can build a workout that is unique to you (see pages 180–9).

You will notice the workouts have no beginner, intermediate or advanced levels – that is on purpose. As a beginner you may struggle to complete the exercises for the whole of the active interval, but don't give up: dig deep and keep trying. We all have to begin somewhere and the only thing you need to remember if you are new to training is that you should start with a lighter-weight kettlebell at first (see What You Will Need, page 20).

Choosing a discipline will be determined by your personal fitness goals. For improvements in *lean muscle mass, muscle strength* and *endurance*, and if you want to *reduce body fat* quickly, look to incorporate one of my **Kettlebell Resistance** workouts.

For *flexibility, strength, endurance* and *speed*, choose a **Bodyweight** workout. You do not need any equipment, just yourself. Great for when you are travelling.

My **Primal Power Stretch** workouts are great if you are looking to increase *flexibility* and introduce *muscle strength* and *core training* to your workouts.

Finally, if you are after a *challenge* and looking to *shake up your training*, hit the **Hero** workouts. I love the body-shock these workouts give me and I'm always totally beat by the end of them!

For those of you who are advanced (and you will all find you progress quickly on this programme once you get into it and as long as you're consistent), you can always leap higher, you can always lift heavier and you can always aim to do one more round in the density finishers!

To recap, the *Your Life – Train for It* rules:

1. Commit to making training a regular, consistent part of your week. Commitment is the real key to bringing about positive results, from finding the time to train, through to challenging yourself to dig deep in the final seconds of your last active interval.

2. Commit to getting started and set some achievable goals with dates attached to them. Goals give you something to aim for and are a vital way to track your fitness progress. See Your Progress, page 20, for ways to get inspired and keep on track.

3. Select your focused workout from pages 142–79.

4. Just commit to start each workout and always complete your warm-up.

5. Hang on in there during each workout with 100% effort! Go for it with the exercises and suck it in during the rest periods.

6. If you complete any exercise or workout blocks with ease, then up the kettlebell weight or opt for the more intense variation of the move. You must aim to get to the point of failure in order to progress your fitness.

7. Stick at it until the rest periods – never, ever quit during the exercise blocks.

8. Do not skip the cool-down, but enjoy the time as you wind down and reward yourself mentally. Nothing beats that feeling of a job well done!

The only thing you need to do now is . . . begin! The journey is on!

4 | EXERCISE LIBRARY

The following section is all about technique and mastering the exercises that make up the workouts. The step-by-step instructions here will teach you how to perform each exercise and there are photographs to help demonstrate start positions, posture alignment, correct technique, variations and advancements.

The exercises are divided up into each training discipline – Kettlebell, Bodyweight and Primal Power Stretch.

'The better your exercise technique, the more effective your workout will be and the faster your body will transform.'

'For me, the correcting of bad habits took longer than learning the new exercises. Even for the most committed and experienced athletes, I can guarantee that some of your exercise form will need minor technique adjustments. The better the form, the harder the exercise, and the quicker you will reach your magic fatigue point. You have to learn to train in a way that makes it hard!

Education is what this chapter is all about, and for ease I've divided it up into sections that reflect my methods of training: Kettlebell Resistance, Bodyweight and Primal Power Stretch. Each section introduces the fundamental exercises, how to do them and the parts of the body you will work whilst performing the exercises.'

UNDERSTANDING THE TERMINOLOGY

Good posture
Posture can be defined as the alignment of your joints and muscles to assist in movement and exercise function. Simply stated, it is the way in which your muscles and skeleton hold your body erect.
We all strive for good posture or good

spinal alignment, not just because it looks aesthetically pleasing but because it can help reduce a number of negative health consequences, such as joint stiffness and back pain. And it keeps the core in focus.

Ultimately, good posture creates a strong and stable spine, which is key to maintaining good spinal health.

When the topic of posture comes up in conversation, people immediately start to suck their stomach in to the extreme, pull back their shoulders to the extreme and try to 'look' taller by lifting their chins to the extreme. But typically when we do this it actually has an adverse effect on good posture.

Here are a few handy points to help obtain good posture and to help you look a little less 'stiff':

■ Stand with your feet a shoulder-width apart, toes pointing forwards and your weight primarily on the balls of your feet.
■ Stand up straight, as if a climbing rope is attached to the top of your head gently pulling upwards.
■ Keep your head neutral and your ears in line with your shoulders.
■ Lift your ribs away from your hip bones and slide your shoulders back and downwards, allowing your arms to stay relaxed and hang naturally at the side of your body.
■ As you exhale, tighten through your abdominals, drawing your navel back and downwards towards your spine.

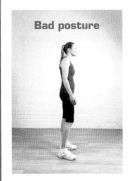
Bad posture

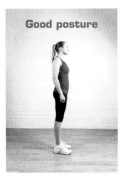
Good posture

Braced abdominals and activating your core tension

Engage, activate, tighten, brace and switch on your abdominals: all these phrases are bandied about when it comes to undertaking any fitness routine; we hear them all the time. If you think about it, do the phrases make sense and, likewise, as exercise practitioners do we truly understand what the cue is actually prompting us to do?

Personally, as a fitness coach I have to admit I use these cues a great deal. Call it old habits. My favourite is 'activate your core tension', and you will see it appearing several times in this chapter. For me it is not really about the words in the phrase, it is more about reminding you to focus on the core.

The first thing to know is that all the workouts that Bear and I have designed develop this core strength and require you to contract your key core muscles in an abdominal brace, so it is worth first understanding a little about your core.

Your core is essentially a complex series of muscles, excluding your arms and legs, that you use in the majority of your daily movement patterns. 'Core stability' is the strength of the muscles that hold the spine and pelvis in place, allowing your limbs to move more freely.

I am not going to go into a long-winded point-by-point dialogue on how to gain the ideal abdominal brace. Instead I am going to give you my quickest and, to date, my most effective way of contracting your key core muscles in an abdominal brace.

Imagine someone is about to punch you directly in your stomach – or, like Bear, you have taken a massive leap off a cliff and are about to land in survival mode.

The instinctive tightening just before you hit the floor, or before the punch is landed, is your core engaging. You are contracting your abdominal brace and activating your core tension. Now, as you exhale, concentrate on holding this contraction. It is this tightening sensation that you will need to activate when you set your core tension.

KETTLEBELL RESISTANCE TRAINING

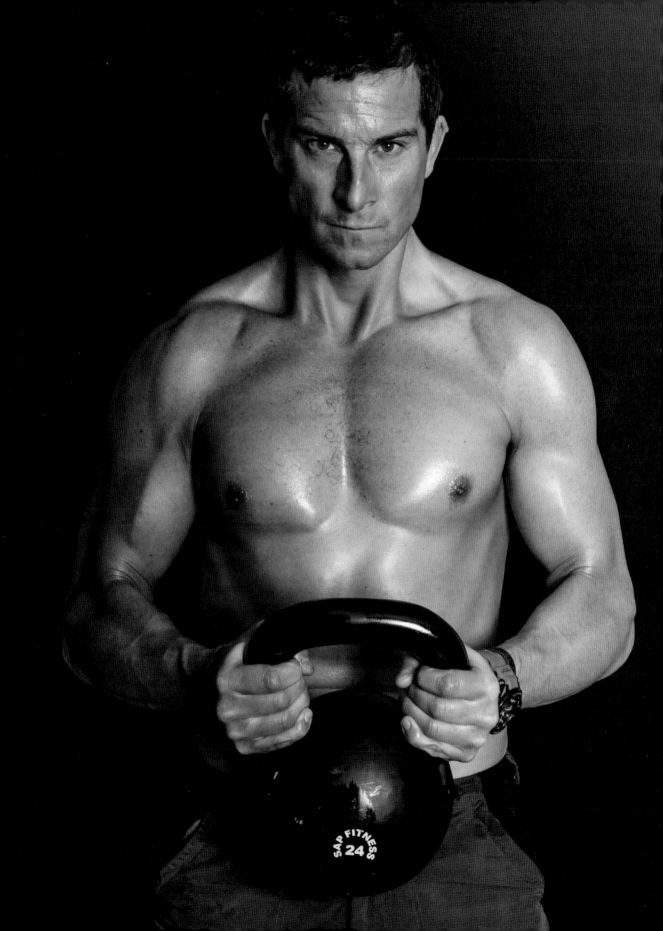

KETTLEBELL GRIPS

When you first begin to train with kettlebells it's worth taking the time to master the various grips used with this equipment. At first it's not uncommon to experience the odd ache in your forearms, but this is often a result of not holding the kettlebell correctly.

Learning the correct grip positions will not only help prevent muscle ache, but will reduce muscle fatigue and injuries to your forearms; it will also help you to master the kettlebell movements properly and so to reap the full benefits of the exercises. To reiterate, take time getting acquainted with the following grip techniques and with handling the kettlebell in general.

Single-hand grip

For a single-hand grip you will pick the kettlebell up in one hand.

- Start with the kettlebell on the floor and reach your hand down towards it, fingertips first.
- Grasp the handle of the kettlebell firmly, with your knuckles facing away from your body.
- Continue to maintain a firm hold on the kettlebell handle in the palm of your hand at all times.

The single-hand grip forms the foundation of many of the kettlebell exercises that you will encounter in your workouts, such as the 'Single-hand Swing' and 'One-arm Kettlebell Row'.

Double-hand grip

For a double-hand grip, you will pick the kettlebell up in two hands using the kettlebell handle.

- Start with the kettlebell on the floor and reach both hands down towards it, fingertips first.
- Grasp the handle of the kettlebell firmly with both hands – your knuckles should be pointing forwards, with your thumbs and index fingers touching.
- Continue to maintain a firm hold on the kettlebell handle in the palms of your hands at all times.

Ball grip

For a ball grip, you will grasp the bell and the horns of the kettlebell with the base facing downwards.

- Start with the kettlebell on the floor and reach both hands down towards it, fingertips first.
- Place your thumbs on the inside around the top part of the kettlebell horns so that your thumbs are pointing away from your body.
- Open the fingers of both hands widely and then clasp them firmly on to the bell of the kettlebell.
- Try to spread your fingers as much as you can so that you are supporting as much of the bell as possible.

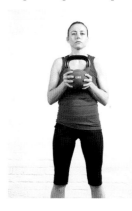

Horn grip, or bottom-up/bottom-down grip

For the kettlebell horn grip ('bottom-up/bottom-down' grip), you will grasp the kettlebell in two hands using the horns, so that your thumbs and index fingers are touching the bell of the kettlebell, with the kettlebell base facing upwards.

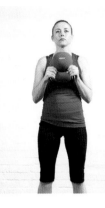

- Start with the kettlebell on the floor and reach both hands down towards it, fingertips first, hinging your wrists at 45 degrees and positioning your thumbs forwards.
- Place both thumbs on the inside of the horns of the kettlebell so that the tips of your thumbs point back towards your body.
- Grasp the outside of the kettlebell horns with your fingers.
- Using your biceps, curl the kettlebell upwards towards your body so that the base is facing upwards and the kettlebell is close to your body.
- Take care when using this grip and always maintain a firm grip on the kettlebell horns.

Regular hand grip

- With a single-hand grip (see page 28), position the kettlebell on the back of your forearm as shown in the photograph.

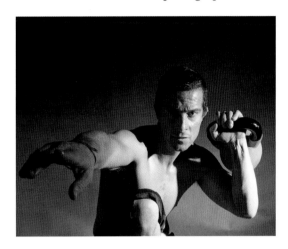

Rack position

- Grip your kettlebell using a regular hand grip (see above) with the handle at 45 degrees at the base of your palm.

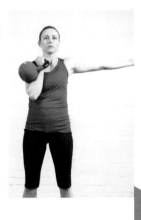

- Hug your hand into your chest and allow the bell of the kettlebell to sit snugly in the crook of your elbow.
- Keep your elbow tucked in and close to the crest of your hip to hold in the rack position.

TIP! It will be more comfortable on your wrist if you remove any jewellery or watches for this grip.

1 | SINGLE-HAND SWING

Target Areas: shoulders, back, hips, glutes and legs. Emphasis: posterior chain, core and legs.

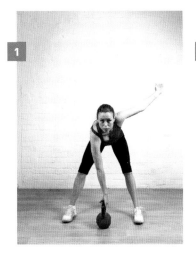

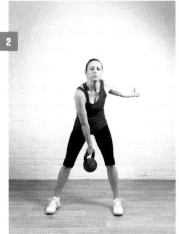

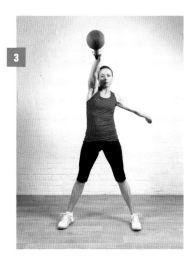

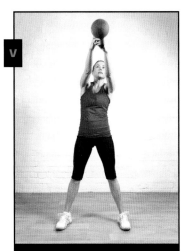

VARIATION:

Try the alternating single-hand swing. As the kettlebell reaches shoulder height switch hands to alternate from one side to the other. Use your hips to drive the move. The less you use your legs, the harder your core has to work.

HOW TO DO IT:

- Stand with your feet a hip-width apart with a kettlebell placed on the floor centrally between your legs, a little forward of your toe line.

- Activate and brace your abdominals. Hinge at your hips and bend your knees to reach for the kettlebell with your right hand. You should feel a slight stretch in the back of your legs and hamstrings as you reach forward to pick up the kettlebell.

- Grab hold of the kettlebell using a single-hand grip (see page 28).

- Keep your chest straight and, for balance, reach out the opposite arm to the side at shoulder height with the palm facing up. Try not to squat too deep.

- Hinge further at your hips to drive the kettlebell backwards between your legs.

- Once the kettlebell passes between your legs, straighten your legs and knees, and squeeze your buttocks to create a thrusting motion, allowing the kettlebell to travel forwards up to shoulder height. Take three short swings to get it up to shoulder height. At shoulder height, the kettlebell should feel weightless.

- As the kettlebell drops back down, hinge at your hips first and then your knees to repeat the motion.

2 | DOUBLE-HAND SWING

Target Areas: back, abdominals, hips, shoulders, glutes and legs. Emphasis: whole body.

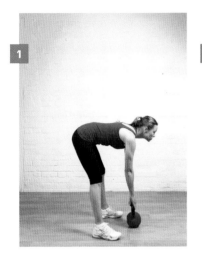

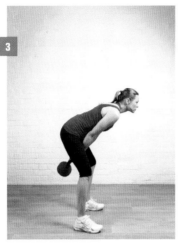

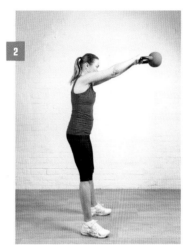

VARIATION:

For added intensity you can swing the kettlebell all the way up to the overhead position. This variation is an advanced move and should only be performed once you are confident with your technique. Stay loose in your arms but keep your grip tight to avoid letting go accidentally.

Make sure you have enough clearance space overhead and choose a lighter kettlebell to start with. Complete a few swings to shoulder height first before extending overhead.

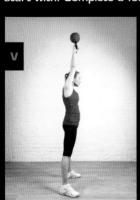

I love this move as it really engages the core and improves balance and power.

HOW TO DO IT:

- Stand with your feet approximately a hip-width apart with the kettlebell placed on the floor centrally between your legs.

- Hinge at your hips first and set your core tension. Bend to pick up the kettlebell using a double-hand grip (see page 28).

- Keep your chest upright and push your hips back to drive the kettlebell backwards between your legs with a slight bend in your knees. Try not to squat too deep.

- Once the kettlebell passes between your legs, squeeze your glutes and, with a thrusting motion, swing the kettlebell forward between your legs and up to shoulder height. At this point, the kettlebell should feel weightless and you have fully extended through your legs and hips.

- As the kettlebell drops back down, hinge at your hips and bend your knees to repeat the motion.

3 | STANDING ABDOMINAL 8s

Target Areas: abdominals, hamstrings and back.   Emphasis: abdominals.

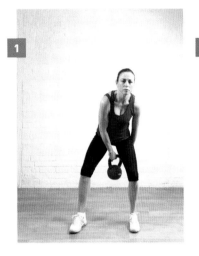

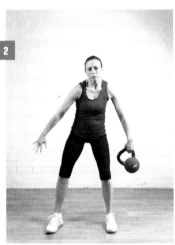

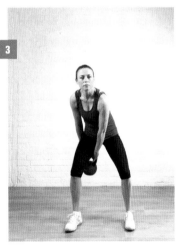

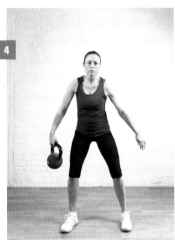

HOW TO DO IT:

- Stand with your legs just slightly wider than a shoulder-width apart with a kettlebell in your right hand, using a single-hand grip (see page 28).

- Push your hips back and bend your knees slightly to stand in a shallow squat position, maintaining an upright chest and straight back.

- Brace your abdominals and keep your chest lifted.

- Pass the kettlebell through the front of your legs and swap hands at the outside of your left leg. Bring the kettlebell around the left leg and then back through to the right leg. Swap hands to make a figure of 8.

- As the kettlebell comes around each leg, squeeze your glutes and stand up straight, snapping your hips forward.

- Repeat the action, continuing to make figures of 8.

TIP! Keep the motion as smooth as possible.

V

VARIATION:

Abdominal 8s to Woodchop

- As you pass the kettlebell around the back of your leg, swap hands and then drive the kettlebell up on to your opposite shoulder, creating a diagonal line of movement.
- Catch the kettlebell in a half ball grip (see page 28).
- Return the kettlebell back through your legs to continue the figure of 8 movement and drive it up to catch on your opposite shoulder.

TIP! When at shoulder height, always keep the kettlebell below chin level.

TIP! Keep your eyes on the kettlebell to ensure it doesn't hit your knee.

4 | KETTLEBELL DEADLIFT

Target Areas: whole body.   Emphasis: hamstrings, glutes and posterior chain in general.

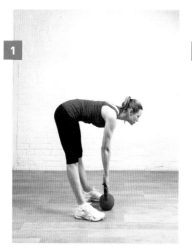
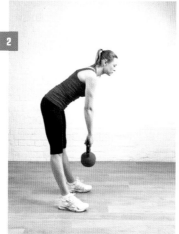
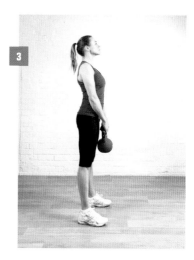

HOW TO DO IT:

- Stand with your feet just slightly wider than a hip-width apart with the kettlebell placed on the floor centrally between your legs. Pull your shoulders back and brace your abdominals.

- Keeping your legs straight, hinge at the hips and pick up the kettlebell using a double-hand grip (see page 28).

- Exhale as you lift and straighten your chest.

- Start to push down through your heels and as you drive your hips forward stand up straight. Keep the kettlebell close to your body.

- Hinge at your hips first, then your knees and, without compromising good spinal alignment, lower the kettlebell back down to the floor to complete the move.

Target Areas: posterior chain, hamstrings and core stabilization. Emphasis: glutes.

HOW TO DO IT:

- Place a kettlebell at the centre of your right foot, just in front of your second toe, and stand with your feet just slightly wider than a hip-width apart.

- Drop your shoulders back and down and shift your weight on to your right leg.

- With a slight bend in your right knee, hinge at your hips and lift your left leg behind you to assume a single-leg stance.

- Keeping a neutral spine position, continue to hinge forward until your upper body and left leg are parallel with the floor.

- Grab the kettlebell using the double-hand grip (see page 28).

- Bring yourself to an upright position, keeping the kettlebell close to your body and holding your single-leg stance.

- With a slight bend in your right knee, hinge at your hips, keeping your left leg behind you in the single-leg stance.

- Keeping a neutral spine position, continue to hinge forward until your upper body and left leg are parallel with the floor. Touch the kettlebell to the floor to complete the move.

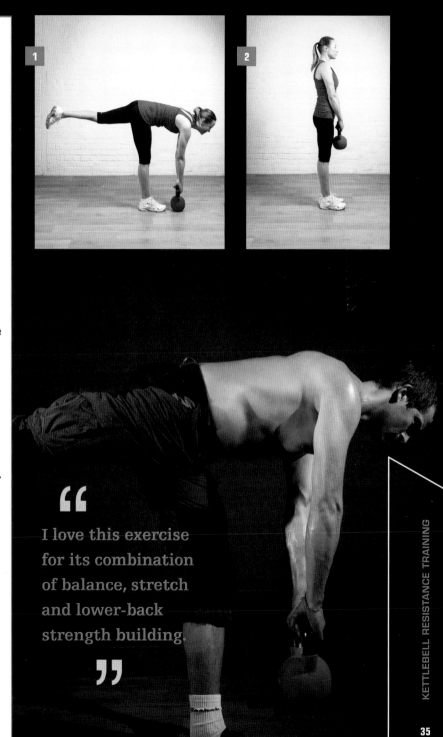

> **I love this exercise for its combination of balance, stretch and lower-back strength building.**

6 | HIP BRIDGE AND KETTLEBELL CHEST PUSH

Target Areas: strengthens stabilization muscles. Emphasis: glutes and abdominals.

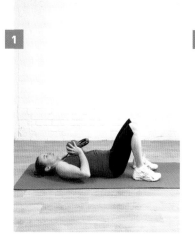

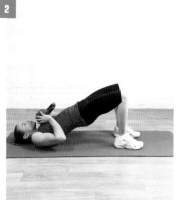

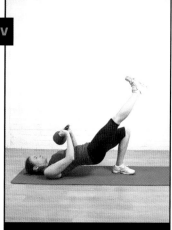

HOW TO DO IT:

- Lie on your back with your knees bent and feet on the floor a hip-width apart.

- Hug the kettlebell close to your chest using the bell or horn grip (see pages 28–9), with your elbows tucked in close to your body.

- Squeeze your glutes and lift your hips off the floor, creating a straight line from your knees to your shoulders.

- Check your shoulders stay in contact with the floor and that your bodyweight is evenly distributed.

- Stay in your Hip Bridge and push the kettlebell away from your chest in a straight line, fully extending your arms.

- With control, lower the kettlebell back to mid-chest and slowly lower your body to the starting position.

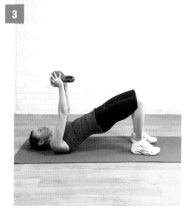

VARIATION:

At the top of the move, lift one leg off the floor. Flex your foot towards your face and press your heel to the ceiling.

7 | HIP BRIDGE PULL-IN

Target Areas: whole body. Emphasis: glutes, core and back.

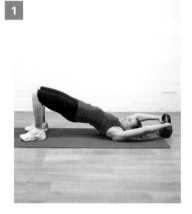
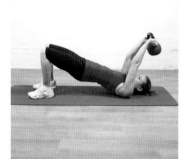
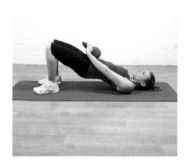

HOW TO DO IT:

- Place a kettlebell at the top of your mat.

- Lie on your back with your knees bent and feet on the floor a hip-width apart.

- Straighten your arms above your head and hold the kettlebell in a bottom-down horn grip (see page 29).

- Squeeze your glutes and lift your hips off the floor. Roll up off the mat, pushing each vertebra into the floor as you rise. At the top of the move there should be a straight line from your knees to your shoulders.

- Ensure that your shoulders stay in contact with the floor and that your bodyweight is evenly distributed to create the Hip Bridge.

- Stay in your Hip Bridge position and, keeping your arms straight, start to lift the kettlebell off the floor in an arc-like motion towards your thighs.

- Slowly and with control, reverse the movement until the kettlebell is back on the floor to complete the movement.

8 | ABDOMINAL PULL-INS

Target Areas: arms and abdominal muscles. Emphasis: abdominals.

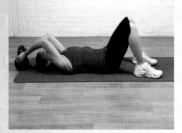

1

HOW TO DO IT:

- Lie on your back with your knees bent and your feet flat on the floor a hip-width apart.

- Place a kettlebell on the floor above your head, holding it in a horn grip position (see page 29), with your elbows pointing upwards towards the ceiling.

- On your exhale, curl up to shorten the gap between your ribs and your hips, simultaneously bringing the kettlebell over your head towards your chest.

- At the top of the movement squeeze your abdominals as you fully exhale.

- Make sure that your elbows are tucked into the sides of your ribs and that your shoulders are lifted off the floor.

- Slowly reverse the movement, curling back down to return the kettlebell to the start position.

TIP! Ensure your lower back stays in contact with the floor throughout the move.

2

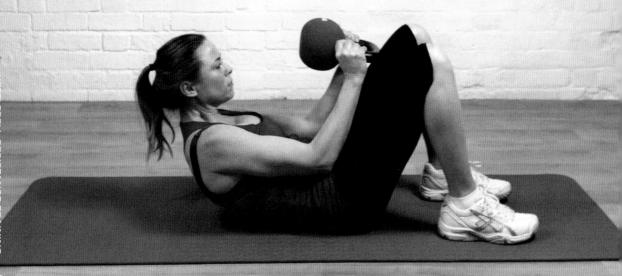

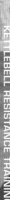

9 | ABDOMINAL CRUNCH TO STANDING

Target Areas: abdominals, shoulders, arms and legs. Emphasis: abdominals and legs.

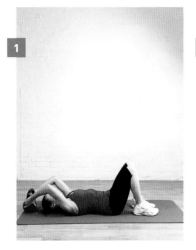
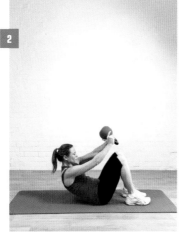
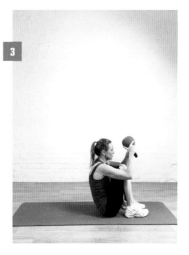

HOW TO DO IT:

- Lie on your back with your knees bent and your feet flat on the floor a hip-width apart.

- Place the kettlebell on the floor above your head and grip it with both hands, using a horn grip (see page 29). Point your elbows upwards towards the ceiling.

- As you exhale, curl up to shorten the gap between your hips and your ribs and simultaneously bring the kettlebell over your head towards your chest.

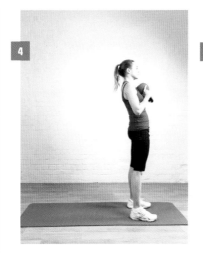
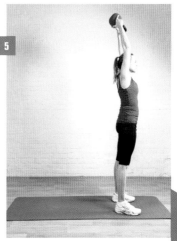

- Continue to curl up and, pressing through both feet, push up to a standing position. Extend your arms to press the kettlebell overhead before lowering it again to your chest.

- Hinge at your hips first, then bend the knees and lower your body until your seat bones find the floor.

- Keeping your feet flat on the floor, roll back until your shoulders are in contact with the floor and your arms and kettlebell are fully extended overhead to complete the move.

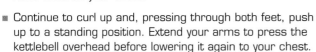

> " This is a favourite exercise as it targets the whole body and requires balance, poise and power. "

Target Areas: back, shoulders, arms and core. Emphasis: middle back.

HOW TO DO IT:

- Stand with your feet a hip-width apart and place a kettlebell centrally between your legs, next to the inside of your ankles. Take a big step back with your right foot in a wide split lunge position.

- Lower your body and deepen the lunge position, making sure your left knee is in direct alignment over your ankle.

- Keep your hips forward as much as possible and turn your right foot out 45 degrees, making sure the outside of this foot stays in contact with the floor.

- Lean forward from the hips.

- With your eye gaze directed towards the inside of your left foot, grab the kettlebell with your right hand, using a single-hand grip (see page 28).

- Brace your abdominals and, with a neutral spine, lift the kettlebell off the floor. Glide your elbow past your ribs in a smooth movement until the kettlebell reaches the top of your hip or just above.

- Lower the kettlebell to the floor to complete the movement.

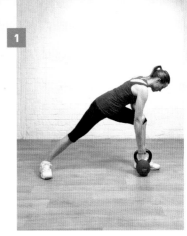

11 | KETTLEBELL POWER PLANK

Target Areas: whole body. Emphasis: core and shoulders.

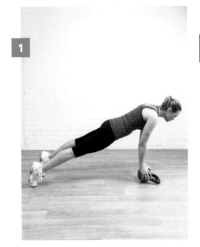

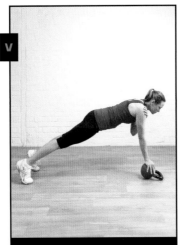

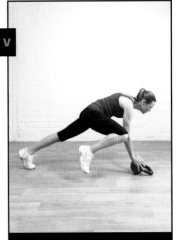

HOW TO DO IT:

- Place a kettlebell centrally at the top of your mat. Drop the hand of the kettlebell towards the top of the mat, away from you, with the bottom of the kettlebell facing towards you.

- From a kneeling position, lean forward and place your hands on the kettlebell in a ball grip (see page 28).

- Straighten your arms and activate your core tension as you tuck your toes under and lift your knees as your come into a High Plank position.

- Squeeze your glutes and focus on maintaining a straight line from your feet to your shoulders to complete the move.

VARIATION:

Kettlebell Single-arm Plank

Start in Kettlebell Power Plank. Slowly lift your left hand off the kettlebell and place it on to your right shoulder. Keep your hips parallel to the floor and maintain a straight line from your feet to your shoulders.

VARIATION:

Kettlebell Spider Plank

Start in Kettlebell Power Plank. Without compromising your alignment, slowly bring your right knee to the outside of your right elbow. With control, return to your starting plank position. Repeat on your left-hand side to complete one repetition.

TIP! For maximum results, keep your nose in front of your fingertips and keep your abdominal tension activated.

KETTLEBELL RESISTANCE TRAINING

12 | KETTLEBELL POWER PLANK WITH ROW

Target Areas: abdominals, arms and back. **Emphasis:** core and back.

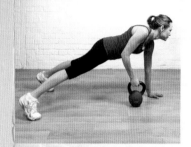

1

HOW TO DO IT:

- Start in High Plank position (see page 41). Place a kettlebell to your right, at mid-chest.

- Engage your abdominals, activate your glutes and focus on maintaining a straight line from your feet to your shoulders.

- Grab the kettlebell firmly using a single-hand grip (see page 28) and raise it off the floor to hip level or just above and hold.

- Keep your weight forward over your shoulders. Lower the kettlebell back down to the floor.

2

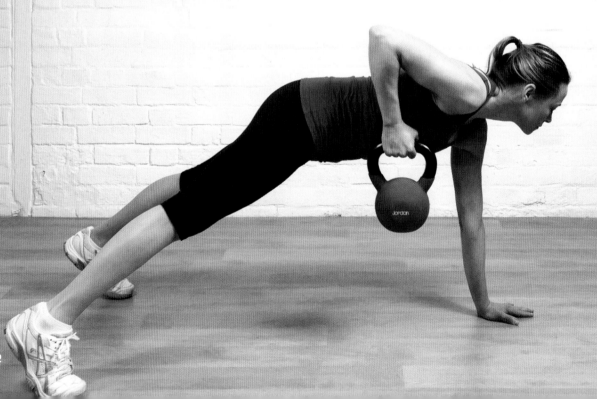

13 | KETTLEBELL POWER PLANK WITH RENEGADE ROW

Target Areas: abdominals, arms and back. Emphasis: core and upper back.

HOW TO DO IT:

- Start in High Plank position (see page 41), with your hands resting on a pair of kettlebells placed directly under your shoulders.

- Activate your core tension and glutes. Concentrate on keeping a straight line from your feet to your shoulders.

- Hold each kettlebell firmly in a single-hand grip (see page 28).

- Lift one kettlebell off the floor towards your shoulder, keeping your weight forward over your shoulders, without twisting or tilting your hips.

- Lower the kettlebell back down to the floor and begin to lift/row the other kettlebell off the floor towards your shoulder, without twisting or tilting your hips.

- Lower the kettlebell back down to complete the move.

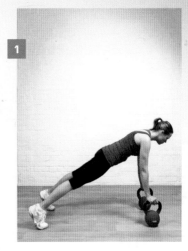

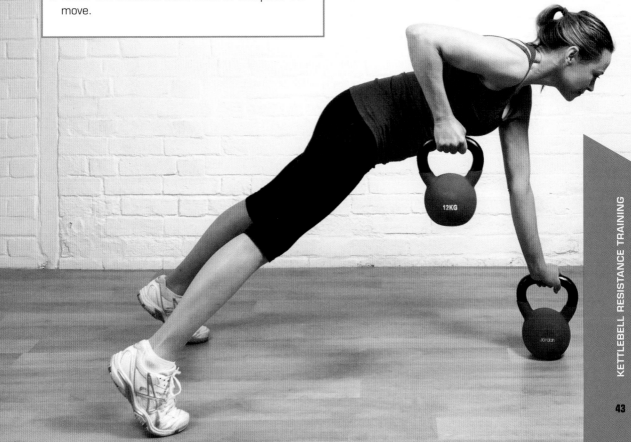

14 | KETTLEBELL FRONT SQUAT

Target Areas: legs, glutes and back.   Emphasis: legs.

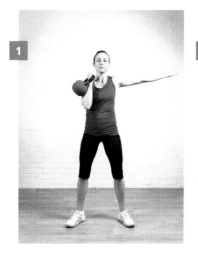

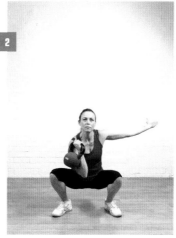

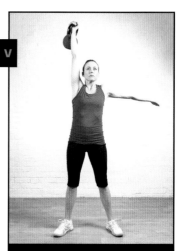

HOW TO DO IT:

- Hold a kettlebell in a rack position on your right arm (see page 29) and stand with feet just slightly wider than a hip-width apart, toes turned slightly outwards.

- Straighten your left arm out to the side at shoulder height, palm facing upwards.

- Hold the kettlebell tightly and keep your right elbow close to your body.

- Drive your hips backwards and bend your knees, keeping your weight on your heels as you lower yourself towards the ground.

- Continue to bend your legs until your thighs are parallel with the ground or just slightly lower.

- Squeeze your inner thighs and keep your chest up as you bring yourself back to the starting position.

VARIATION:

Kettlebell Front Squat to Press **At the bottom of the Front Squat position begin to drive upwards and simultaneously extend your arm and press the kettlebell in an overhead position. Slowly return the kettlebell down to the rack position and as above to begin the movement again.**

TIP! Keep your weight evenly distributed as you drive through your heels to rise out of your low squat position.

15 | GOBLET SQUAT

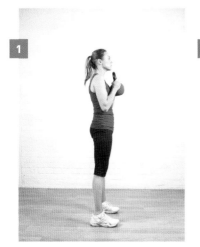

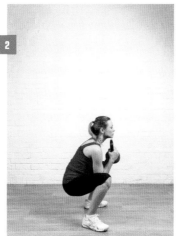

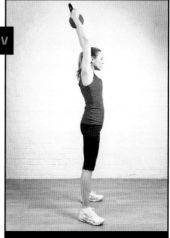

HOW TO DO IT:

- Stand with your feet just slightly wider than a hip-width apart, with your toes turned slightly outwards.

- Hold a kettlebell in a ball grip (see page 28) close to the chest, with your elbows tucked into your ribs.

- Hinge at your hips first and push your buttocks back until your thighs are parallel to the ground or just slightly lower, then bend your knees to start the squat.

- Continue to go deep into the squat, aiming to drop your hips below your knees, keeping your chest upright and taking care not to compromise good spinal alignment. Keep your eye gaze forward.

- At the bottom of the squat, use your elbows to gently push your knees outwards. Drive through your heels to bring yourself back up to standing, squeezing through your glutes at the top of the squat.

VARIATION:

Goblet Squat and Press
At the bottom of the Goblet Squat position begin to drive upwards and simultaneously extend your arms to press the kettlebell up into an overhead position. Slowly return the kettlebell down to the start, as above, to begin the movement again.

KETTLEBELL RESISTANCE TRAINING

16 | TWO-ARM KETTLEBELL MILITARY PRESS

Target Areas: **shoulders, arms and back.** Emphasis: **shoulders.**

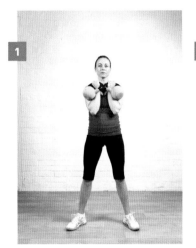 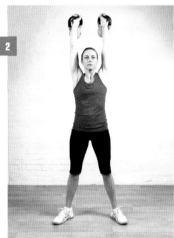 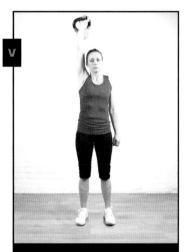

HOW TO DO IT:

- Hold one kettlebell in each hand in a rack position (see page 29), elbows tucked in close to your ribs.

- Brace your abdominals and, with a slight forward lean at the waist, press the kettlebells upwards until your arms are fully extended.

- Press your chest forward through your arms, keeping your chin parallel to the floor.

- Bring the kettlebells back down to your starting position to complete the move.

TIP! Keep your wrists straight as you press the kettlebells upwards to complete the overhead press.

VARIATION:

Single-arm Kettlebell Military Press

- Hold a kettlebell in your right hand in a rack position (see page 29). Keep your right elbow tucked in close to your ribs.

- Activate your abdominal tension and press the kettlebell upwards until your right arm is fully extended.

- Keep your arm close to your ear and your chin parallel with the floor.

- Slowly bring the kettlebell back down to the starting rack position to complete the move.

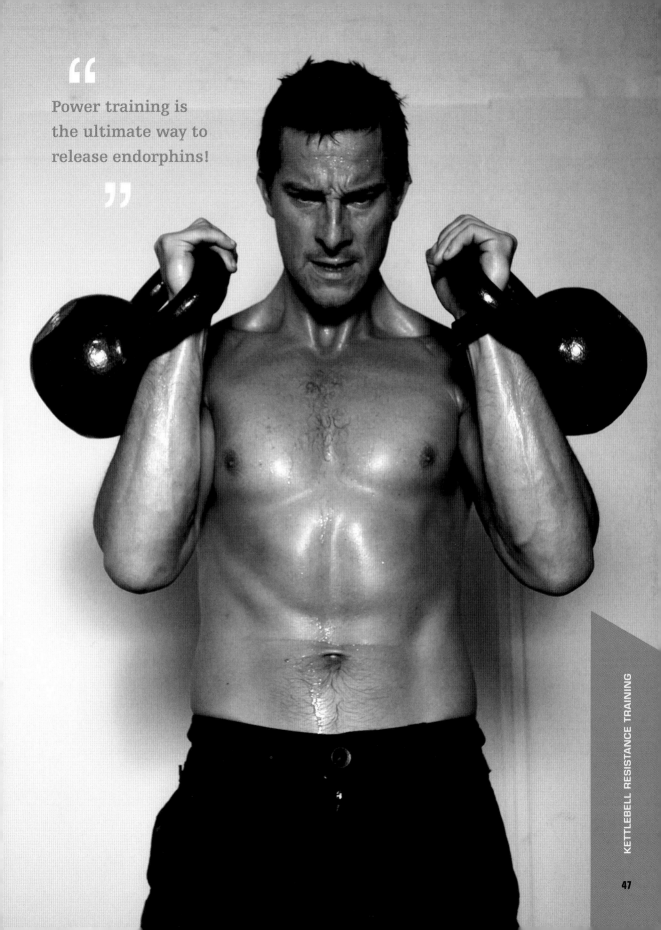

> "Power training is the ultimate way to release endorphins!"

17 | KETTLEBELL LUNGE AND PRESS

Target Areas: quads, hamstrings, glutes, shoulders, triceps.

HOW TO DO IT:

- Stand up straight holding a kettlebell in a rack position (see page 29) on your right side, feet just slightly wider than a hip-width apart.

- Take a big step backwards with your left foot into a high split lunge position with your left arm out at your side.

- Bend your right knee towards the floor to deepen the lunge and simultaneously press the kettlebell up overhead, extending your arm fully and keeping your elbow tucked in, so that it tracks close to your body's mid-line. Your arm should be extended straight behind your ear, with the kettlebell resting on the back of your arm in a regular grip.

- Keep your hips and shoulders facing forward throughout the move and your right knee aligned directly above your ankle.

- Press the ball of your left foot into the floor and rise up out of the lunge. At the same time, bring the kettlebell back down to the starting rack position.

TIP! If you are alternating legs with this workout, use an alternating single-hand swing (see page 30) to change sides.

18 | BICEP TO DOUBLE-HAND MILITARY PRESS

Target Areas: arms, shoulders, abdominals and back. **Emphasis:** arms and shoulders.

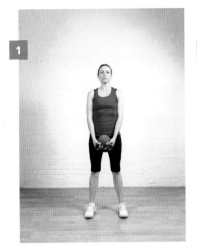
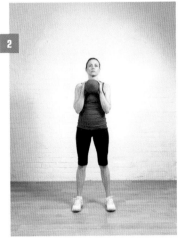
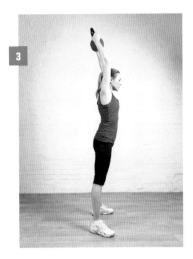

HOW TO DO IT:

- Stand with feet a hip-width apart, holding a kettlebell at hip level using a ball grip (see page 28), with arms fully extended.

- Keep your elbows close to the body and curl the kettlebell up towards your chest until you reach the full range of movement. Pause at the top.

- Slowly extend your arms fully overhead and drop your shoulders away from your ears.

- Press your chest forwards through your arms, squeezing your shoulder blades together to allow your arms to pass just behind your ears, lifting your chin to keep it parallel to the ground.

- Carefully lower the kettlebell and return it to the top of the bicep curl position.

- Curl the kettlebell back down to your hips to complete the movement.

19 | KETTLEBELL CHEST PRESS

Target Areas: upper body.   Emphasis: chest.

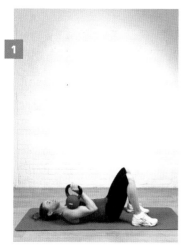

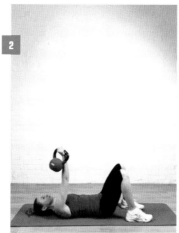

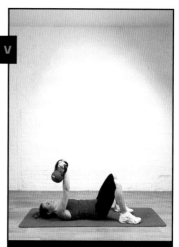

HOW TO DO IT:

- Lie on the floor holding a kettlebell in one hand using a single-hand grip (see page 28).

- Keep your arm bent and your elbow close to your body at mid-chest level.

- Press the kettlebell towards the ceiling in a straight line, fully extending your arm.

- Pause and, with control, bring the kettlebell back down towards your chest to return to the starting position.

TIP! Maintain a good kettlebell grip position and try not to let your elbows flare out to the side as you push the kettlebell away from you.

VARIATION:

Hold one kettlebell in each hand using the single-hand grip (see page 28). Press both kettlebells towards the ceiling either simultaneously, or alternate between right and left extensions.

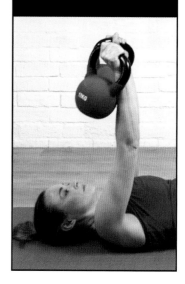

20 | KETTLEBELL WINDMILL

Target Areas: shoulders, back, abdominals, obliques and hips. Emphasis: core.

HOW TO DO IT:

- Stand with your feet a shoulder-width apart with both feet pointing left in a partial block position, at approximately 45 degrees. Hold the kettlebell in rack position (see page 29) in your right arm.

- Press the kettlebell overhead and straighten your arm into the fully extended position.

- Keep your arm close to your ear and your eye gaze on the kettlebell overhead.

- Push your hips and glutes out towards your right arm. Place your left hand on your left leg, with your palm facing out.

- Shift your weight backwards slightly and, with control, lower your upper torso towards the ground, sliding your left arm down your leg as far as possible. Keep your right arm holding the kettlebell straight and directly overhead. Your left leg should also be straight.

- Pause and then reverse the motion back up to your start position.

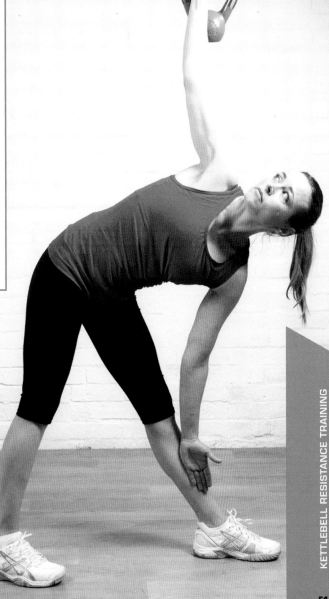

1

2

| **KETTLEBELL DIAMOND PUSH-UPS**

Target Areas: whole body. Emphasis: shoulders, abdominals, chest and triceps.

HOW TO DO IT:

- Start in High Plank position (see page 41) with a kettlebell placed just in front of you. Place your hands on top of the kettlebell in a ball grip (see page 28).

- Engage your abdominals and make sure your nose is further forward than your hands.

- Flare your elbows out to the side and lower yourself towards the ground.

- Once your elbows are bent at 90 degrees or slightly less, start to push your body back up to the start position.

- Keep your core stabilization muscles activated to maintain good spine alignment throughout the move.

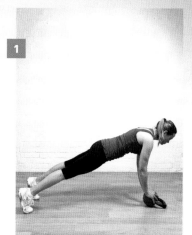

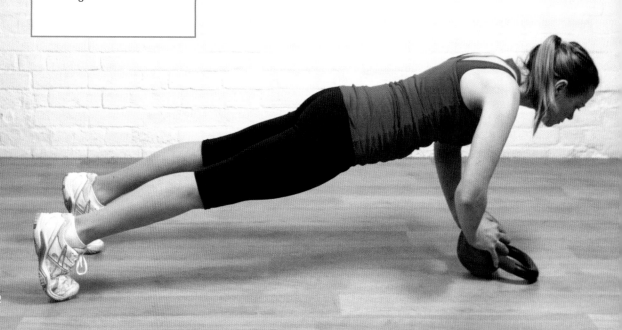

22 | KETTLEBELL POWER PUSH-UPS

Target Areas: upper body and core. Emphasis: chest.

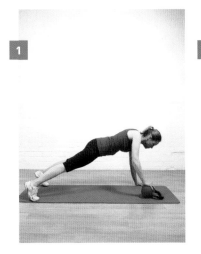

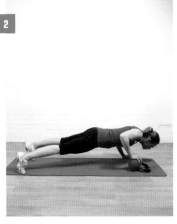

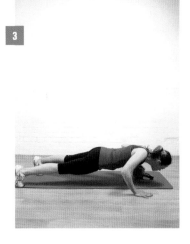

HOW TO DO IT:

- From High Plank position (see page 41), place your right hand on top of the kettlebell at mid-chest and your left hand on the floor a shoulder-width apart.

- Engage your abdominals and lower your body until your arms are at 90 degrees.

- Push your body off the floor, and release your hands from the floor and from the kettlebell to perform an upper-body power jump.

- At the same time as you push off the floor, leap to the right and, as you return to the floor, land your left hand on the kettlebell and your right hand on the floor a shoulder-width apart to complete the move.

- Keep your core tension and don't compromise your back position throughout the move.

> " A great fundamental move that I love! The ability to leap your whole body off the ground and land with precision is a handy tool for a survivor. This move helps build great dynamic power and eye-to-hand coordination when jumping or grabbing things in the wild at speed! "

Target Areas: obliques, arms and core stabilization muscles. **Emphasis:** oblique abdominals.

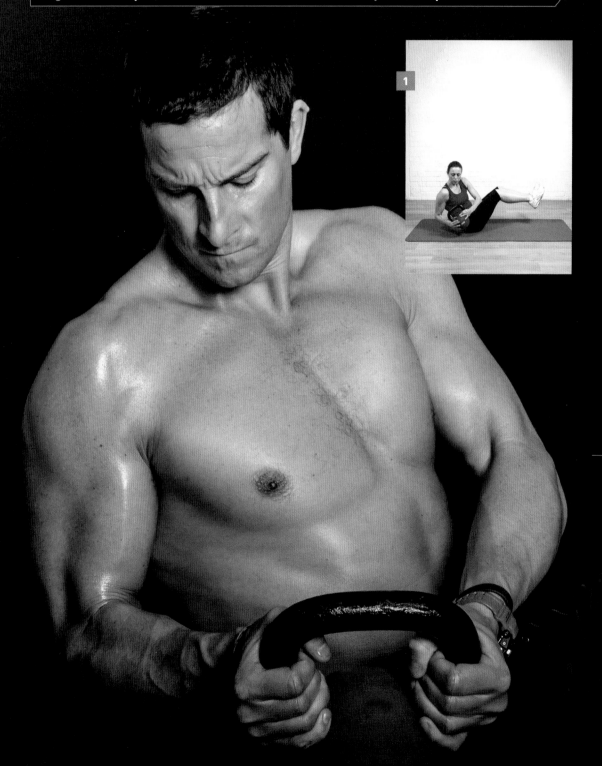

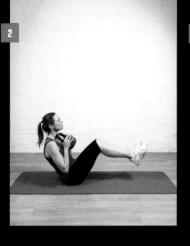

2

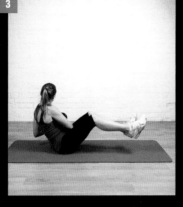

3

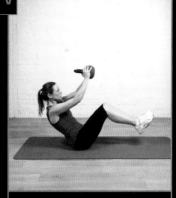

V

HOW TO DO IT:

- Sit on the floor with a kettlebell positioned to your right-hand side by your hips. Bend your knees and place your feet flat on the floor.

- Keep your spine straight and lean back until you feel your abdominals start to engage.

- Slowly lift both feet off the floor and push your knees together to help keep your balance.

- Pick up the kettlebell with a double-hand grip (see page 28) and pass it up and across your body, rotating through your torso. Ensure you twist your upper body only, keeping your lower body still and in place.

- Tap the kettlebell to the floor on your left, then reverse the action and continue tapping from side to side to complete the movement.

TIP! Keep your neck lengthened throughout movement and check your weight is distributed evenly across your buttocks.

VARIATION:

Bear Twist and Press

As you lift the kettlebell from one side to the other, pause momentarily as the kettlebell comes to mid-chest. Extend your arms to press the kettlebell up and away from you. Bring the kettlebell back to mid-chest and continue with the Bear twist.

24 | KETTLEBELL 3-POINT RUSSIAN TWIST

Target Areas: abdominals, arms and core. Emphasis: obliques.

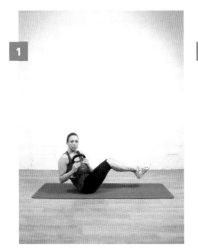

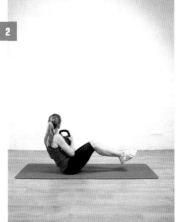

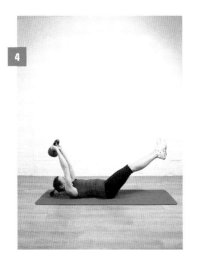

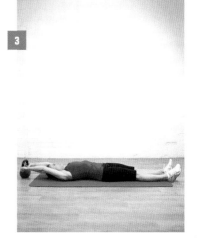

HOW TO DO IT:

- Place a kettlebell next to your right hip and sit upright on the floor with your knees bent and your feet flat on the floor.

- Keeping your back straight, slowly lean back until you activate core tension.

- Grab the kettlebell in both hands, holding it in a horn grip with the base facing down (see page 29).

- Lift both feet off the floor and grip the knees together to balance.

- Move the kettlebell from the right side of your body to the left side, twisting through your torso. Keep your hips and legs still.

- When the kettlebell has reached the other side of your body, tap it on the floor.

- Bring the kettlebell to mid-chest position and extend your arms upwards, bringing the kettlebell overhead.

- Stretch out, bringing your body to the floor and extending your legs out straight.

- Raise your legs, then bend your knees into your chest and simultaneously bring the kettlebell back to mid-chest as you crunch and return to your seated position to complete the move.

25 | TURKISH GET-UP HALF

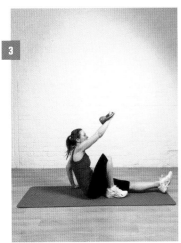

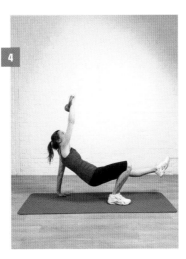

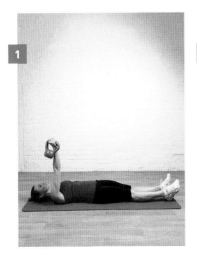

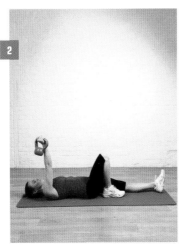

HOW TO DO IT:

- Lie completely flat on the floor. Place a kettlebell to the right-hand side of your chest, within reach.

- Take hold of the kettlebell in your right hand using a regular grip (see page 29).

- Extend your right arm straight up towards the ceiling, with your knuckles pointing towards your head. Keep your eye gaze firmly on the kettlebell for the whole move.

- Bend your right knee and keep your foot flat on the floor. Brace your abdominals.

- Press your left forearm into the floor and begin to roll up to a seated position.

- From the seated position, and supporting yourself on your extended left arm, begin to lift your bodyweight off the floor and into a hover position.

- Pause and reverse the motion to return to the start position to complete the movement.

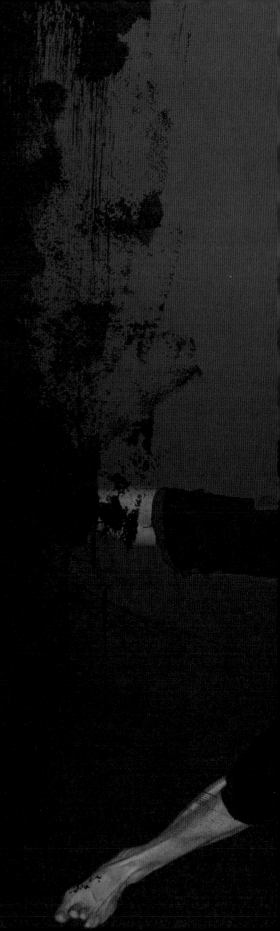

BODYWEIGHT TRAINING

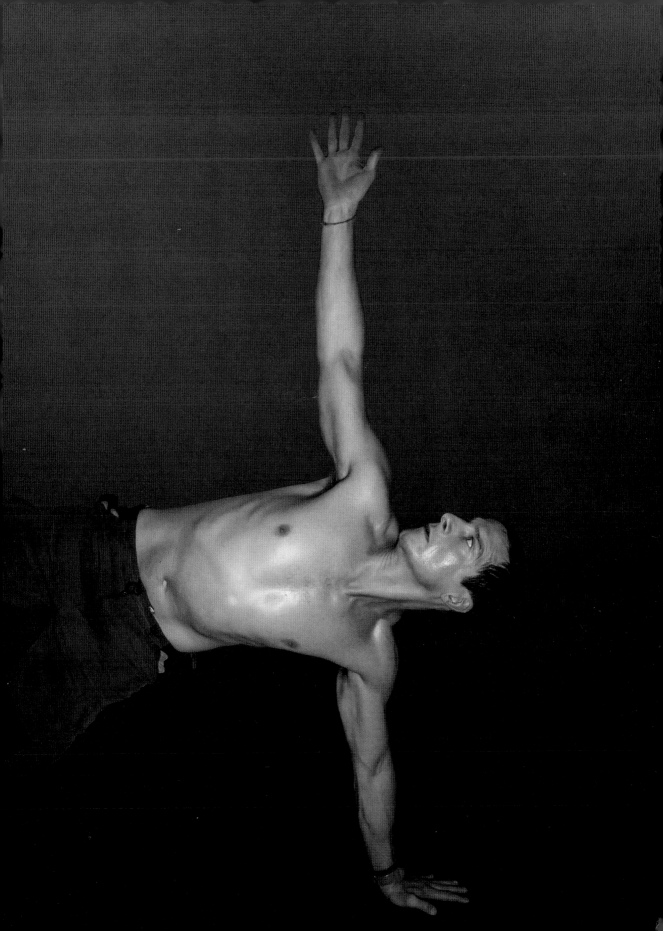

1 | LOW PLANK

Target Areas: whole body. Emphasis: core.

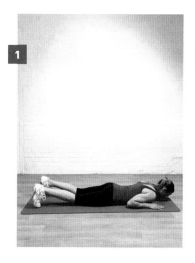

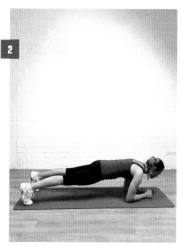

TIP! Ensure that your hips don't rise up and that your tummy doesn't drop down. Keep your thighs, glutes and core engaged through the move. This is all about maintaining your mid-line. Epic abdominals start with an awesome plank.

HOW TO DO IT:

- Lie face down on the floor and rest your body on your forearms. Keep your chin tucked in and drop your shoulders away from your ears.

- Activate your glutes, brace your abs and push off your forearms and toes to lift your body off the floor until your hips are parallel with your shoulders.

- Maintain a straight line from your head to your feet to complete the move.

2 | CRAWL PLANK

Target Areas: whole body. Emphasis: coordination and core stabilization muscles.

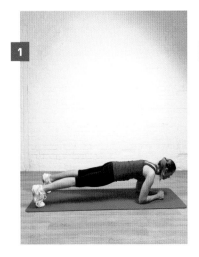
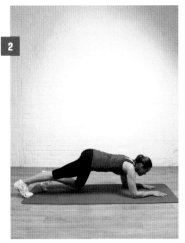
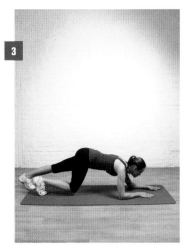

HOW TO DO IT:

- From Low Plank position (see page 60), contract your abdominals and move your right arm and left leg forward by an inch.

- Your body should form a straight line from your shoulders to your ankles at all times, with minimal or no twisting at your hips.

- Pause and move your opposite arm and leg forward so that you start to move forwards across the floor.

'I am here to condition your body and mind. To turn your soft flesh into hard muscle, your weak will into iron resolve.'

Commando Physical Training Instructor

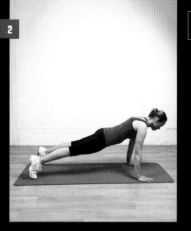

1

2

V

VARIATION:

High to Low Planks

Alternate between High Plank and Low Plank. Be careful not to twist too much through your hips and go for quality over quantity or speed.

HOW TO DO IT:

- Start in Low Plank position (see page 60).

- Keeping a neutral spine alignment, push up off your forearms and come up on to your hands (one at a time).

- Continue to brace through your abdominals, and gently lift your knees and activate your thighs.

- Tighten through your glutes and slide your shoulders away from your ears, with your eye gaze towards the floor.

- Maintain a straight line from your head to your shoulders to complete the move.

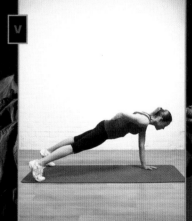

V

VARIATION:

Single-hand Plank

From High Plank position, raise one hand off the floor. Keep your hips parallel to the floor, your core strong and your weight forward as you gently place the hand of the raised arm on to the small of your back or stretched out in front of you.

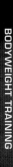

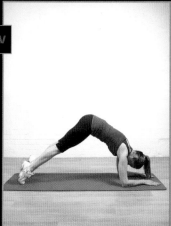
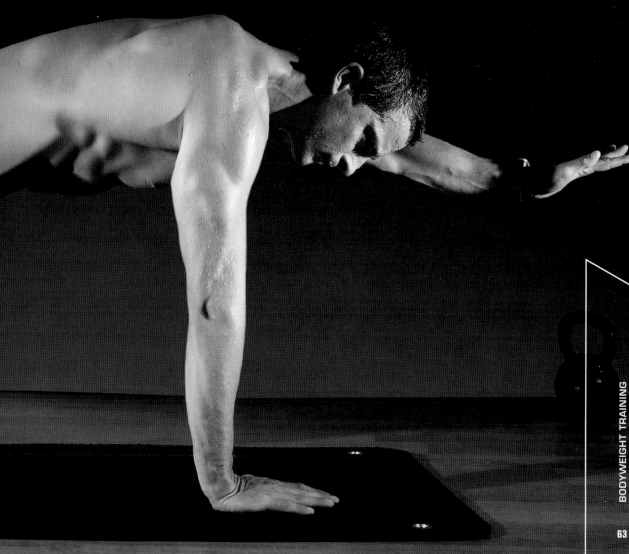

4 | SPIDER SIDE PLANK

Target Areas: whole body. Emphasis: coordination, core stabilization muscles and obliques.

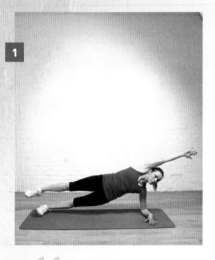

1

HOW TO DO IT:

- Lie on your left-hand side, with your upper body propped up on your elbow and your legs straight. Make sure your elbow is positioned directly under your shoulder and your hips are stacked on top of each other.

- Tighten through your abdominals and elevate your hips off the floor to create a straight line from your shoulders to your ankles.

- Extend your right arm overhead and keep it in line with your ear, eye gaze forward.

- Squeeze your glutes, lift up your right leg and slowly bring your right elbow and knee together to perform a side crunch.

- Fully extend your leg and arm in between repetitions, without lowering your lifted leg.

"
Strong, powerful obliques help to act as a shock absorber – vital protection for your ribcage against any direct impact.
"

2

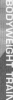

5 | MOUNTAIN CLIMBERS

Target Areas: whole body.   Emphasis: upper body and core.

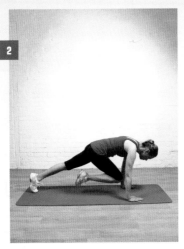

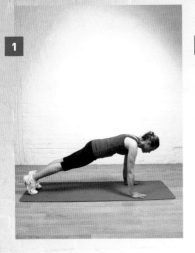

HOW TO DO IT:

- Start in High Plank position (see page 62) and walk your hands out slightly wider than a shoulder-width apart.

- Engage your abdominals. Keep your weight forward and bring your right knee into your chest at speed.

- As you push your right leg back to the start position, quickly bring your left knee in. Continue to alternate your legs.

" This is a key core exercise that I love and throw into almost all my workouts as a great dynamic 'filler' exercise! "

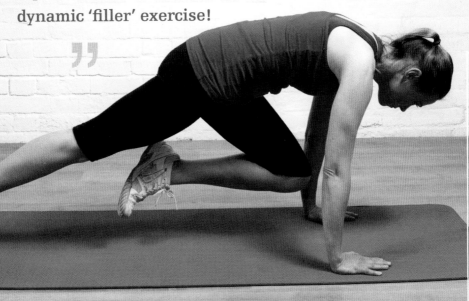

6 | CROSS MOUNTAIN CLIMBERS WITH PUSH-UP

Target Areas: whole body. Emphasis: chest and obliques.

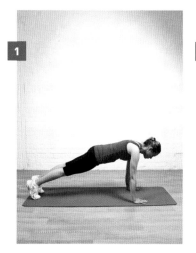

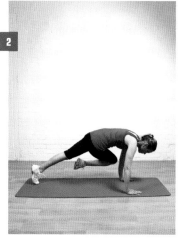

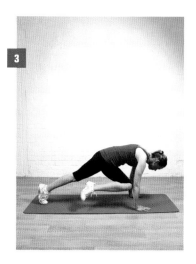

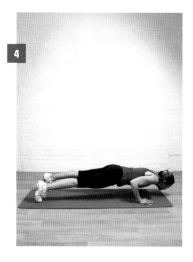

HOW TO DO IT:

- Start in High Plank position (see page 62) and walk your hands out to slightly wider than a shoulder-width apart.

- Engage your abdominals. Keep your weight forward and quickly bring your right knee to the inside of your left elbow.

- As you push your right leg back to the start position, quickly bring your left knee in towards the inside of your right elbow.

- Bend your elbows at 90 degrees and lower your body to the floor. Push your body back up to complete the move.

7 | BEAR LEAP AND REACH

Target Areas: whole body.   Emphasis: shoulders and legs.

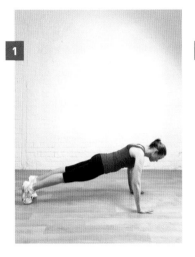

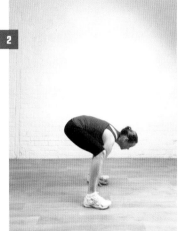

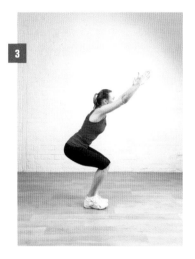

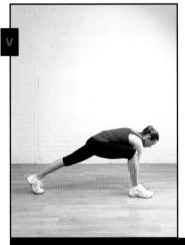

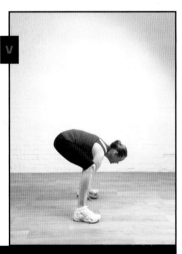

VARIATION:

Walk-in Bear Leap (no jump) **To reduce the impact of the Bear Leap and Reach, start in High Plank position and step your feet to the outside of your hands, one foot at a time. To complete the move, walk or step your feet back to your start position.**

HOW TO DO IT:

- Start in High Plank position (see page 62) with your hands in line and a shoulder-width apart.

- Keeping your hands on the floor, jump forward to bring both your feet to the outsides of your hands. Land in a crouched position with your toes facing forward, your hips low and your elbows close to the insides of your knees.

- Drop lower into your squat, lift your chest up and extend your arms upwards as you reach forward.

- Bring your hands back to the floor. Tip your weight forward into your hands and take a big leap back, landing in a strong High Plank position.

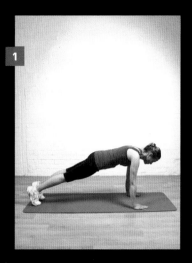
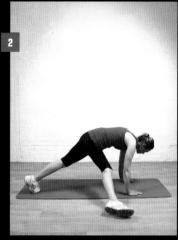
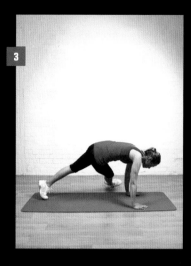

TIP! Rotate your body only slightly in this move. The subtle shift in bodyweight activates more muscle fibre, making it a great whole body exercise!

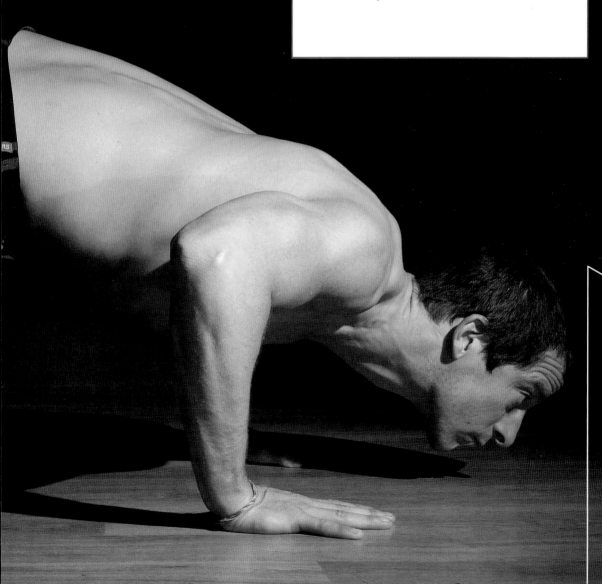

HOW TO DO IT:

- Start in High Plank position (see page 62) and walk your hands out slightly wider than a shoulder-width apart.

- Engage your abdominals.

- Keep your weight forward and bring your left foot diagonally across to your right hand.

- Alternate by 'hopping' your right foot to your left hand to complete the move.

9 | INCHWORM

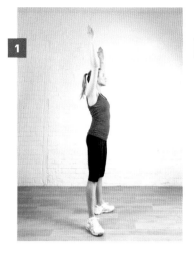

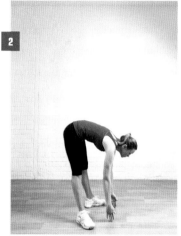

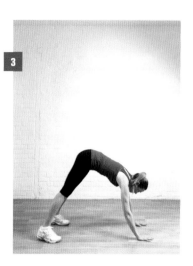

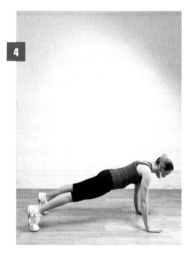

HOW TO DO IT:

- Stand with a good posture, feet a hip-width apart, and extend your arms straight up overhead, with your fingers pointing upwards and palms facing inwards.

- Drop your shoulders back and down, engage your abdominals and hinge forward at your hips, keeping your back straight and arms in line with your ears.

- Continue to hinge at your hips until your hands meet the floor, then walk your hands forward into High Plank position (see page 62). Shift your weight forward so that your nose is forward of your fingertips.

- You can have a slight bend in the knee, but try not to compromise your straight back.

- Walk your hands back towards your feet, keeping your legs as straight as possible to feel a stretch in the back of your legs.

- Bring yourself back up to standing to complete the move.

Target Areas: abdominals, core. Emphasis: abdominals.

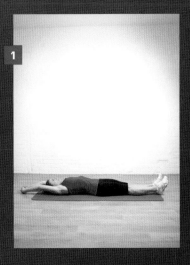

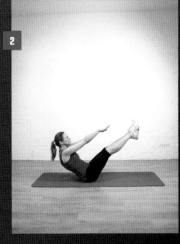

HOW TO DO IT:

- Lie flat on the floor with your arms extended overhead.

- Activate your core tension.

- Bend at the waist and simultaneously start to bring your legs and upper body off the floor.

- Continue to rise up until your hands and feet touch.

- Slowly and with control lower both your legs and your upper body back down to the floor to the start position.

"
I love this sit-up – it gets you to fatigue mega-quick!
"

BODYWEIGHT TRAINING

11 | CROSS CRUNCHES

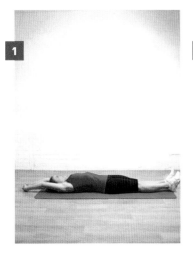
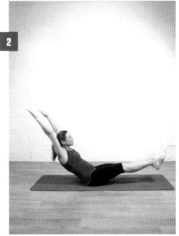
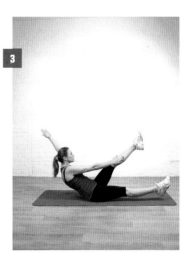

HOW TO DO IT:

- Lie flat on the floor with your arms extended overhead.

- Activate your core tension.

- Bend at the waist and simultaneously start to bring your legs and upper body off the floor.

- Continue to rise up until both your upper body and your legs are at 45 degrees.

- Slowly and under control lower your right leg and lift your left leg to 90 degrees.

- Reach your right arm up diagonally and crunch up to tap the outside of your left ankle, keeping your legs straight.

- Repeat on the opposite side to complete the move.

> Double the set to challenge yourself. Aarrghh . . . feel that burn!

12 | RUSSIAN TWISTS

Target Areas: core stabilization and abdominals. Emphasis: oblique abdominals.

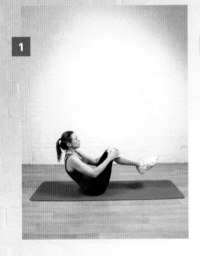

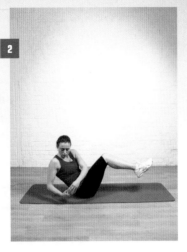

HOW TO DO IT:

- Sit down with your feet flat on the floor in front of you, hands on your knees.

- Keep your back straight and lean back until you feel your abdominals start to engage.

- Slowly lift both feet off the floor and press your knees together to keep your balance.

- Place one hand on top of the other at chest height. Keeping your hips and legs still, twist your upper torso to your right-hand side.

- Aim to tap your right elbow on the floor behind you, as close to your mid-line as possible.

- Keeping your hips and legs still, twist your upper torso to your left-hand side and tap your elbow behind again to complete the move.

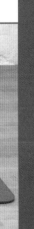

13 | ABDOMINAL ROCK

Target Areas: core and abdominal. Emphasis: core.

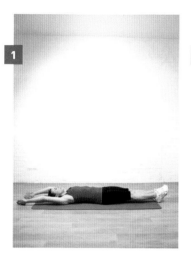

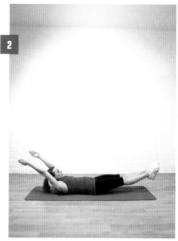

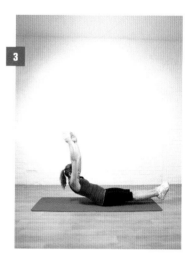

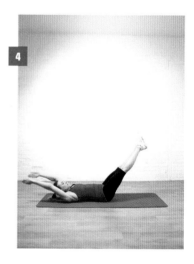

HOW TO DO IT:

- Lie flat on the floor with your arms extended overhead and your legs straight.

- Activate your core tension.

- Bend at the waist and bring your arms and legs off the floor until you feel your abdominals tighten. Your shoulders and feet are now off the floor.

- Gently rock with a forwards and backwards movement, but making sure you do not break core tension, that your abdominals do not create a dome in your tummy and that you keep your arms extended and in line with your ears.

- Continue to rock for the programmed term to complete the move.

“

I find that people have rarely done this exercise before but once they get the hang of it then it's a real ab-burner!

”

14 | ICE SKATERS

Target Areas: lower body, core, arms and coordination. Emphasis: legs.

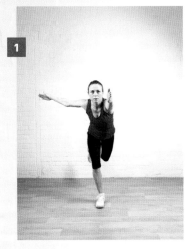

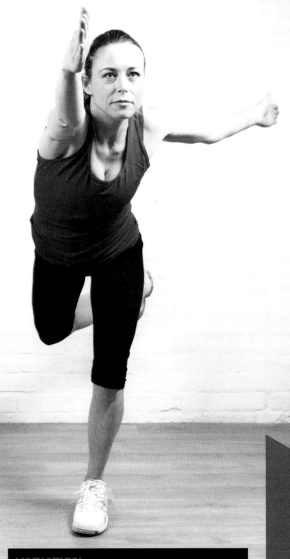

HOW TO DO IT:

- Stand on your right leg with your right knee slightly bent. Bend your left leg behind you with your left knee at 90 degrees.

- Raise your arms to shoulder height, extending your left arm in front of you and your right arm sideways so that your arms are at 90 degrees to each other. Bend your right knee to deepen your stance and then step or leap sideways from your right leg on to your left leg. At the same time switch your arm position, moving your right arm in front of you and your left arm out to the side.

- Keep your chest up and shoulders down.

VARIATION:

Power Ice Skaters **To advance the move, leap higher, wider and bend your legs more so that you can touch to the floor with your hands.**

15 | HIGH KNEES

Target Areas: whole body.   Emphasis: lower abdominals and legs.

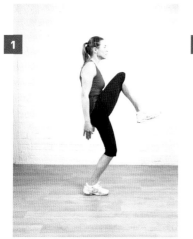

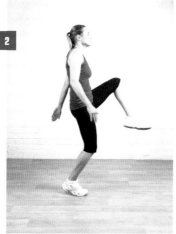

VARIATION:

Move your arms as if you were reaching up and climbing a rope or pulling down a jungle vine.

HOW TO DO IT:

- Stand with a good posture, feet approximately a hip-width apart.
- Lean back slightly and lift your right knee up higher than hip level, towards your chest.
- As you lower your foot to the ground, start to bring your left knee up high past hip level, towards the chest.
- Speed up as you alternate your legs, and lift them as high as you can.

FITNESS TEST

This is one of my core training moves, as it builds speed, power, coordination and flexibility. Go for speed and height.

Challenge yourself to a time trial. How long can you do this move for at speed?

16 | PRIMAL LATERAL LUNGE

Target Areas: whole lower body. Emphasis: legs.

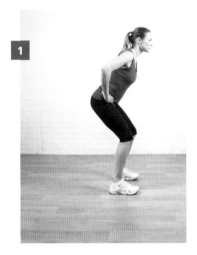
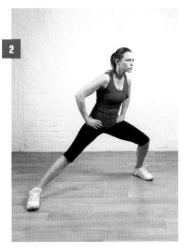
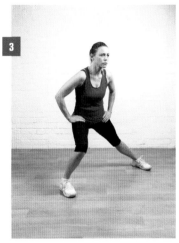

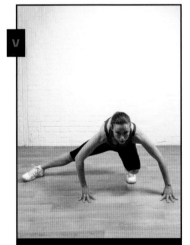

VARIATION:

Start with your hands on the floor and in a low leap position, then complete the lateral lunge as above but keeping your hands on the floor throughout the move.

HOW TO DO IT:

- Stand with a good posture with your feet together and your hands on your hips. Squeeze your thighs together and push your bottom backwards as if you were about to sit down on a chair.

- Hinge further at your hips, bend your knees and lower yourself into a deep squat.

- Brace your abdominals, lift your chest and extend your right leg out wide to your right. Keep your supporting leg bent. Pause.

- Bring your right leg back in and extend your left leg out wide. Keep your supporting leg bent.

- Bring your left leg back to the centre to complete the move.

BODYWEIGHT TRAINING

17 | PISTOL SQUATS

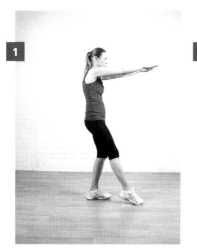
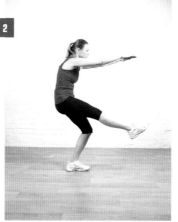
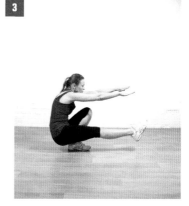

HOW TO DO IT:

- Stand with your feet a hip-width apart, eyes facing forward. Engage your abdominals.

- Hold your arms straight out in front of your body at shoulder height, parallel to the floor.

- Lift your right leg approximately one foot off the floor and hold.

- Hinge at your hips, pushing them back, and lower your body towards the floor.

- Continue to lower as far as you can, keeping your right leg off the floor. Use a wall or post for support as you begin to practice advancing the move.

- Pause long enough to regain your balance, briefly touching the floor with your fingertips, if necessary.

- Start to bring your body back to the starting position without lowering your right leg to complete the move.

BODYWEIGHT TRAINING

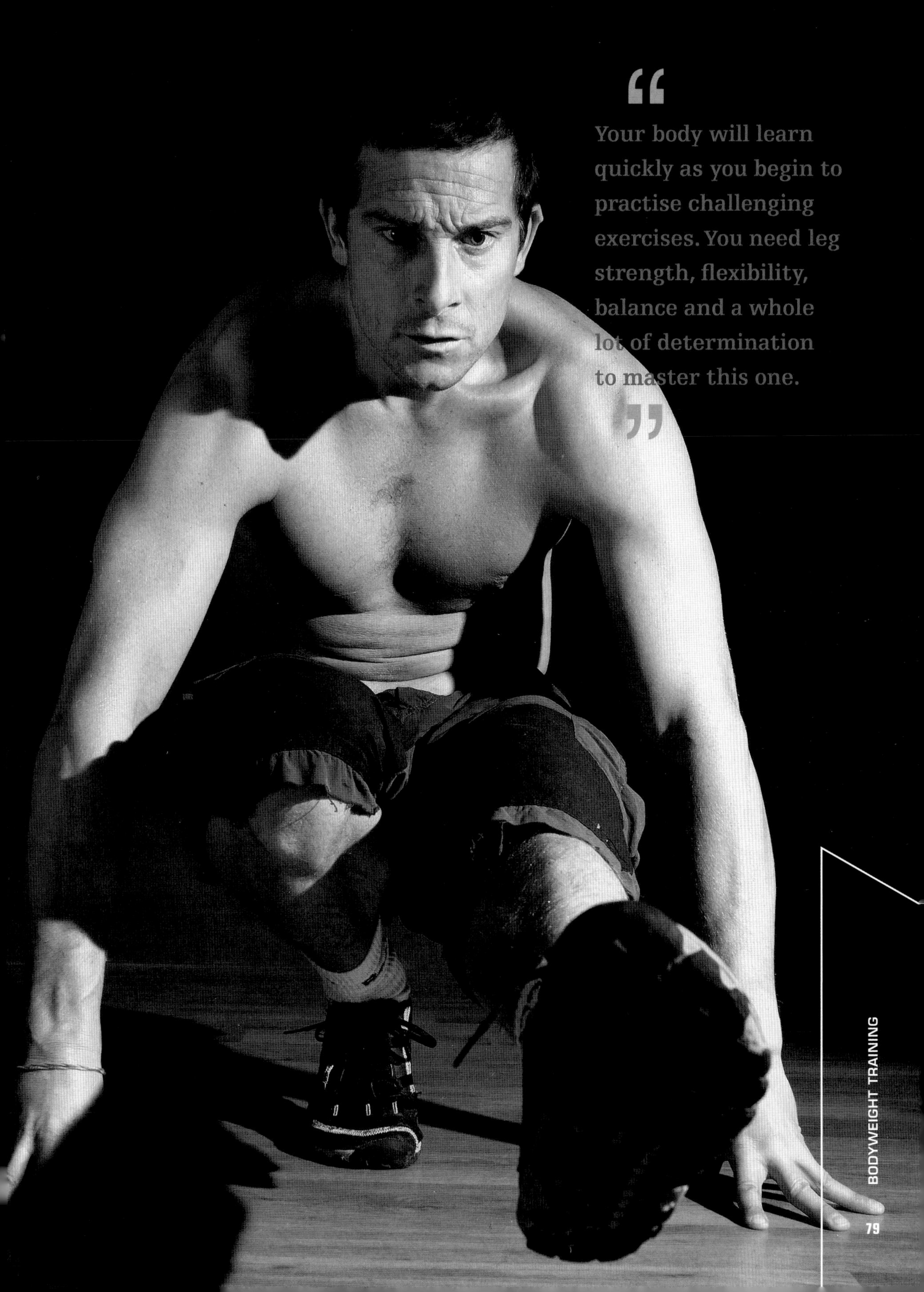

"

Your body will learn quickly as you begin to practise challenging exercises. You need leg strength, flexibility, balance and a whole lot of determination to master this one.

"

18 | SQUAT WITH ARMS

Target Areas: legs, back, abdominals and arms. Emphasis: legs.

HOW TO DO IT:

- Stand with your feet a shoulder-width apart, with your arms extended overhead. Pull your shoulders back and down.

- Brace your abdominals.

- Begin to hinge at the hips first and then bend the knees. Keep your eye gaze forward and your arms in line with your ears.

- Lower your body as far as possible without compromising your neutral spine or your arm position.

- Continue to lower your body until your thighs are parallel to the floor or just below.

- Press through the balls of your feet and squeeze your inner thighs to return to the starting position.

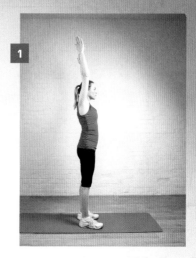

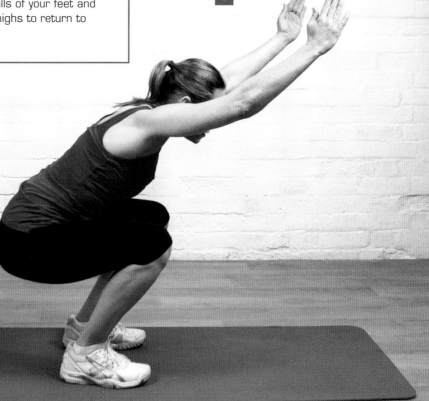

19 | SQUAT TO ABDOMINAL ROLL-OUT TO STANDING

Target Areas: whole body. Emphasis: legs and abdominals.

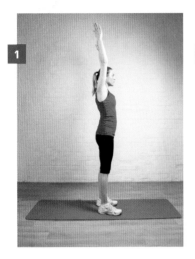

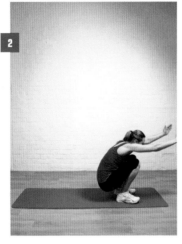

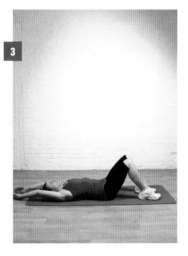

HOW TO DO IT:

- Stand with your feet a shoulder-width apart, with your arms fully extended overhead.

- Keep your eye gaze forward, arms in line with your ears and brace your abdominals.

- Hinge at your hips first, then bend your knees and lower your body until your buttocks find the floor.

- Keeping your feet flat on the floor, roll back until your shoulders are in contact with the floor and your arms are fully extended overhead.

- Reverse the motion to complete the move.

TIP! Keep your heels close to your buttocks as you press your body from a seated position to standing.

Target Areas: legs, back, abdominals and arms. Emphasis: legs and lower abdominals.

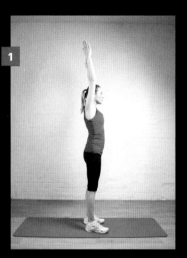

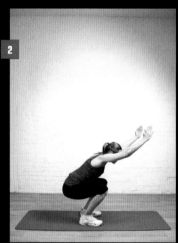

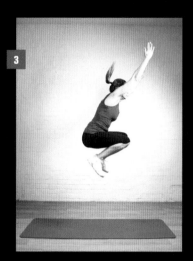

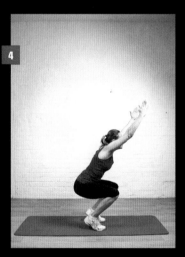

HOW TO DO IT:

- Stand with your feet a shoulder-width apart, with your arms extended overhead.

- Brace your abdominals.

- Begin to hinge at your hips first and then bend your knees. Keep your eye gaze forward and your arms in line with your ears.

- Lower your body as far as possible without compromising neutral spinal alignment or arm position.

- Once your thighs are parallel to the floor or just below, press your heels to the floor and leap up so that your feet leave the floor.

- As you leap up, bring your knees up towards your chest.

- Land lightly in a low squat to complete the move.

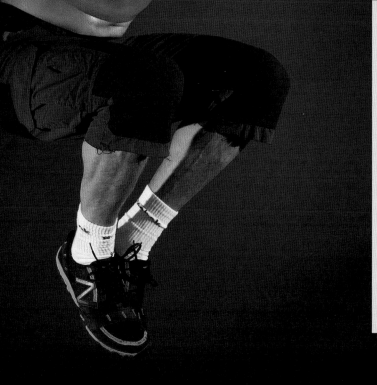

TIP! Go low to get height and lift. Keep your knees soft as you land. I call it the stealth landing!

By adding this small jump at the top of the basic squat exercise you engage your calf muscles and increase your dynamic power and agility.

21 | BEAR TUCKS

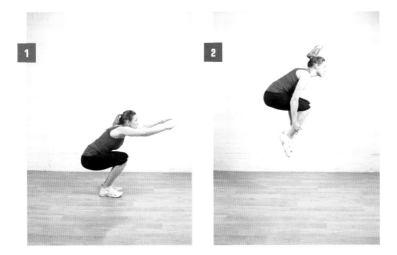

HOW TO DO IT:

- Stand up straight and activate your core tension, with your feet just wider than hip-width apart.

- Extend your arms out in front at chest height.

- Drop into a low squat position and as you hit the bottom of your squat immediately explode upwards off the floor into a jump, bringing your knees up in front and into your chest.

- Re-extend your legs as you return to the floor and land lightly, making sure you absorb the impact as you land with bent knees to complete the move.

> "
> This exercise is a sure-fire way to feel the burn really quickly. It's a killer on the quads and calves as well as being great for cardio. And it builds dynamic power like few other exercises!
> "

22 | HIP BRIDGE DIPS

Target Areas: glutes, hamstrings, lower back and abdominals.
Emphasis: glutes. Improves core and spinal stabilization.

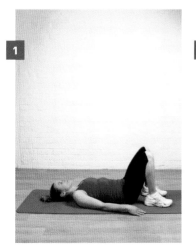

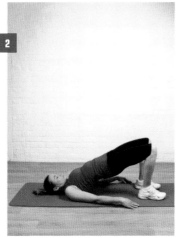

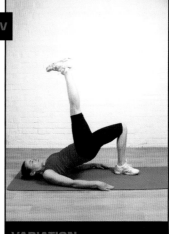

HOW TO DO IT:

- Lie flat on the floor on your back, knees bent and feet flat on the floor a hip-width apart, with your arms at your side, palms down.

- Squeezing through your glutes, lift your hips high into the air, keeping your shoulders on the floor.

- With control, roll down slowly, pressing your mid-back and then your lower back into the floor to return to the start position.

VARIATION:

To advance the move, raise one leg into the air at the top of the move. To further advance the move, keep one leg lifted as you complete your hip dip.

23 | BURPEES

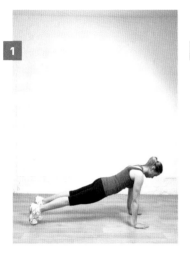

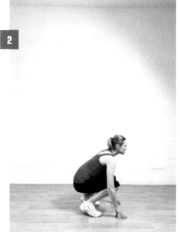

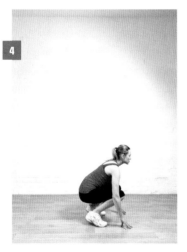

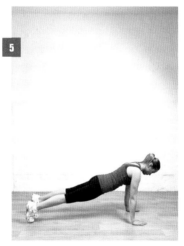

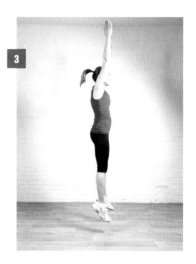

HOW TO DO IT:

- Start in High Plank position (see page 62) with good spine alignment from your hips to your shoulders.

- Set your feet a hip-width apart and, keeping your hands where they are, jump forward to bring your feet between your hands so that you are in a crouch position.

- Leap up into the air with arms fully extended overhead.

- As you land, drop back down into the crouch position, bringing your hands to the floor.

- Keep your hands where they are and spring both feet backwards into the High Plank starting position.

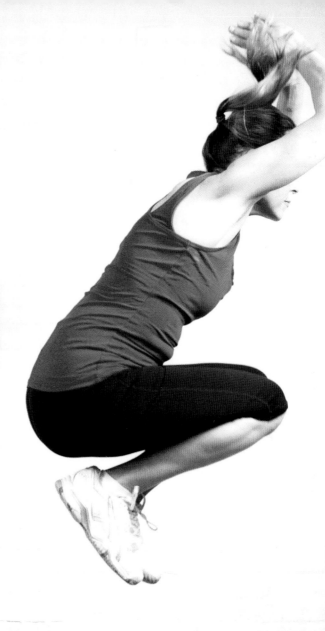

VARIATIONS:

Without leaps Step into the crouch position and then stand up maintaining good posture.

With jump Advance the move even further by leaping up straight into a tuck jump or star jump.

TIP! Great burpees activate major muscle groups, increasing your strength and endurance, and improving your flexibility and tone. Learn to love them as much as the results they give!

“

This is the ultimate workout for spine strength and flexibility which, for me, after my injuries, has been a great one to have developed. In the wild, where I am always encountering rough terrain and have to deal with unexpected impact, this exercise has helped me so much. It has stretched and strengthened my core, legs, back and shoulders.

The crew I film with love this exercise and I can almost guarantee you won't have seen anyone doing this in any gym! That's why I love it – it's a challenge but amazing.

”

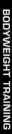

24 | REVERSE PUSH-UP

Target Areas: whole body conditioning. Emphasis: triceps, shoulders and back.

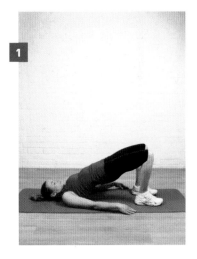

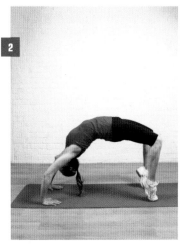

HOW TO DO IT:

- Start in Hip Bridge position (see page 85). Place your hands next to your ears, palms down and fingers pointing towards your toes.

- Press your hands into the floor and push your hips upwards, lifting your body off the floor, arching your spine and engaging your glutes, core and leg muscles.

- Lift both heels off the floor and push up through your chest.

- Pause to feel a full stretch, then slowly lower back down into bridge position and then all the way to the floor.

TIP! Make sure you can hold your Hip Bridge position for 20 seconds before moving on to the full Reverse Push-up.

25 | PULL-UPS

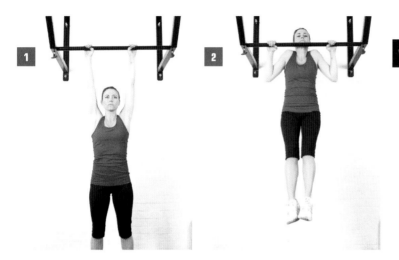

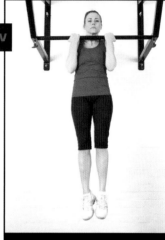

HOW TO DO IT:

- Stand approximately one foot back from a pull-up bar or solid horizontal tree branch.

- Jump up on to the bar with an overhand grip, bracing through your abdominals, with your torso and legs suspended.

- Walk your hands out to approximately one and a half shoulder-widths apart.

- Bending at the elbows, gently pull your body up towards the bar, keeping your legs straight.

- Continue to pull your body up until your chin is over the bar.

- Pause and, with control, gently lower your body back down to the start position.

VARIATION:

Narrow Pull-up **Jump up on to the bar or branch using an underhand grip instead of overhand, and keep your hands just a shoulder-width apart. Complete the exercise as above.**

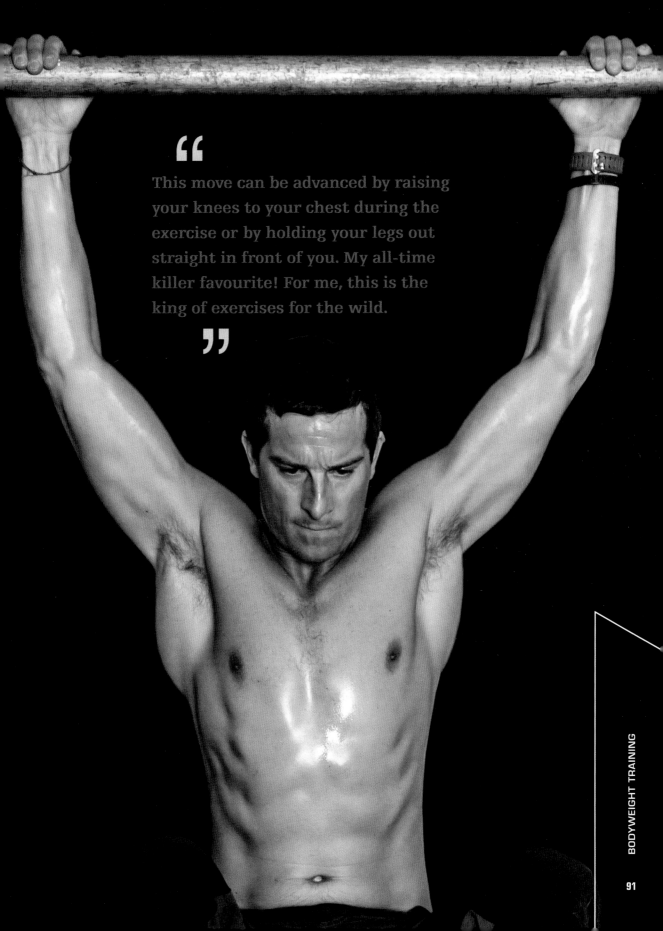

"

This move can be advanced by raising your knees to your chest during the exercise or by holding your legs out straight in front of you. My all-time killer favourite! For me, this is the king of exercises for the wild.

"

26 | HANGING LEG RAISES

Target Areas: whole body.   Emphasis: lower abdominals.

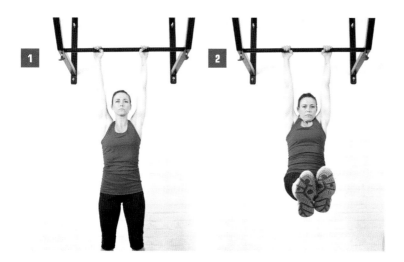

1

2

HOW TO DO IT:

- Stand approximately one foot back from a pull-up bar or solid horizontal tree branch.

- Jump up on to the bar with an overhand grip, bracing through your abdominals, with your torso and legs suspended.

- Walk your hands in to approximately hip-width apart.

- Activate your shoulders and create a tension through your upper body.

- Slowly bring your legs up to 90 degrees, keeping them straight, if possible. Continue to bring them up until they are parallel to the floor.

- Pause and, with control, gently lower your legs back down to the start position.

27 | TOES TO BAR

Target Areas: abdominals, arms, shoulders, back and core. Emphasis: abdominals and hips.

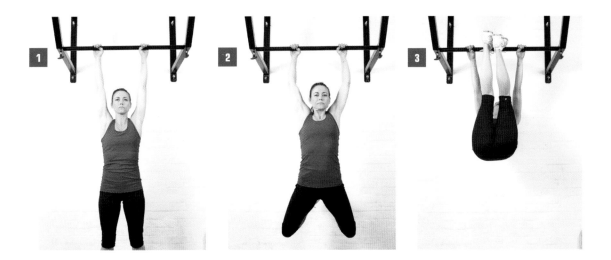

HOW TO DO IT:

- Find a safe bar, tree or stable scaffold to hang from!

- Jump upwards and grab the bar/tree using an overhand grip, with your hands a shoulder-width apart.

- Engage your abdominals and your shoulders.

- Start to bring your feet back up behind you.

- Slowly swing your feet forwards and drive them up towards the bar, bending at the waist.

- Continue to drive your feet upwards towards the bar until your toes on both feet are on the bar.

- Bring your feet all the way down to the start position to complete the move.

This has to be one of my all-time favourite exercises! You can do it anywhere, just as long as you find a safe place to hang. Personally, I always love doing this on the small Welsh island where we live for part of the year. As part of my daily workout there, I use a scaffold pole placed horizontally across a rock gully above a sea cave. (Good motivation to keep hanging on!)

28 | PUSH-UP

Target Areas: whole body. Emphasis: chest and core.

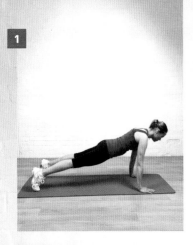

1

HOW TO DO IT:

- Start in High Plank position (see page 62) and walk your hands out to one and a half shoulder-widths apart and in line with your chest.

- Activate your core tension and lower your body towards the floor until your elbows are at 90 degrees or below.

- Keep your back straight, your ears, shoulders and hips in alignment and press through the palms of your hands as you push back up to the start position to complete the move.

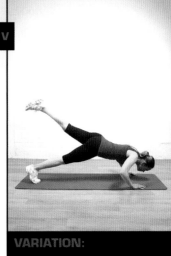

V

VARIATION:

Single Leg Push-up
To advance the move, keep one leg raised off the floor throughout the movement.

2

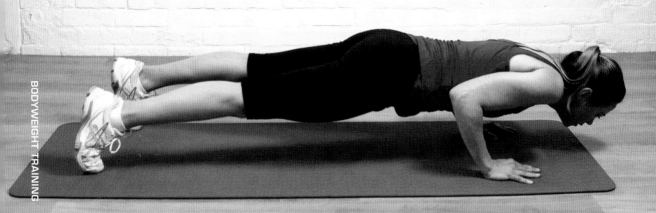

29 | DRAGON PUSH-UP

Target Areas: whole body conditioning and coordination.   **Emphasis:** core, shoulders, arms and chest.

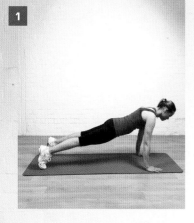

1

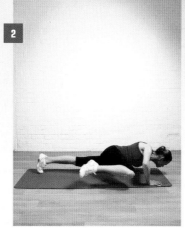

2

3

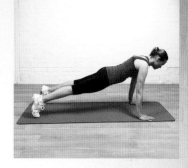

4

HOW TO DO IT:

- Start in High Plank position (see page 62) with your hands slightly wider than a shoulder-width and level with your chest.

- Stagger your right arm slightly forward and bring your right knee out to the side and to your right elbow as you drop down into a push-up. Pause.

- Push up out of the position, returning your right leg to the start position.

- Bring your left hand slightly forward. Bring your left knee to your left elbow as you drop down into the push-up. Pause.

- Push up out of the position, and return your left leg to the start position.

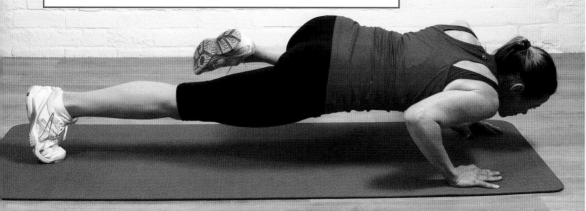

30 | SUPERMAN RAISES

Target Areas: back, core, arms and glutes. Emphasis: core stabilization muscles.

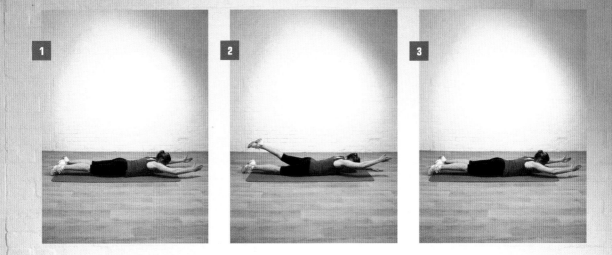

HOW TO DO IT:

- Lie face down on the floor with your chin tucked in and your eye gaze down. Extend your arms out in front into a Superman position.

- Relax your body and, as you inhale, squeeze your glutes and raise your right arm and left leg off the floor.

- Pause at the top of the movement before, with control, slowly lowering your arm and leg to the starting position.

- At the bottom of the movement, inhale and lift your opposite arm and leg off the floor.

- Pause at the top of the movement and, with control, lower slowly to the starting position to complete the move.

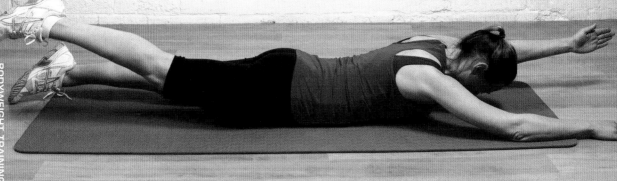

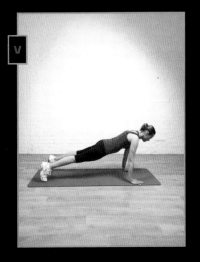

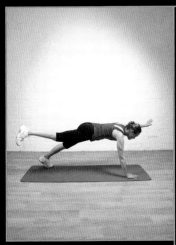

VARIATION:

High Plank Superman

■ Start in High Plank position (see page 62) with your shoulders positioned directly above your wrists. Engage your abdominals and squeeze your glutes.

■ Raise your opposite arm and leg until your arm is level with your ear and your leg at hip height.

■ Pause and hold until you are steady in the position and then slowly return to High Plank position.

■ Repeat on the opposite side to complete the move.

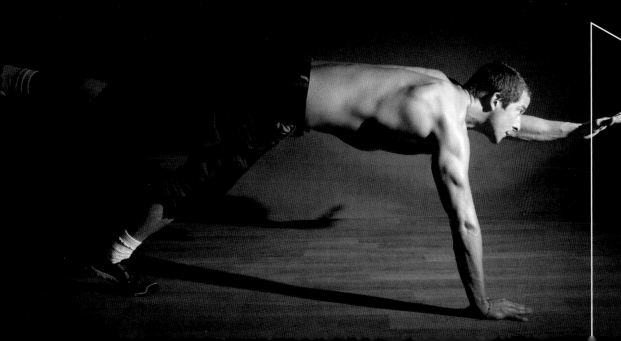

BODYWEIGHT TRAINING

31 | TRI TO SUPERMAN PUSH

Target Areas: whole body, shoulders, arms, core and back. Emphasis: triceps and core abdominals.

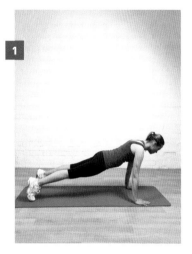

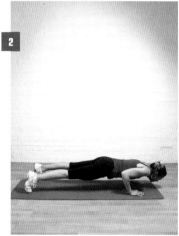

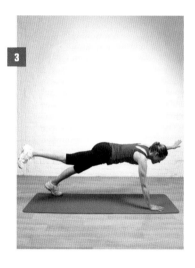

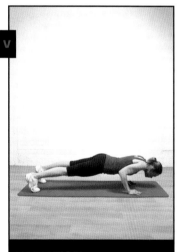

VARIATION:

Narrow Push-up **From High Plank position lower your body until your elbows are bent at 90 degrees. Keep your elbows close to your body as you do this. As you push back up to your start position, keep your core tension activated.**

HOW TO DO IT:

- Start in High Plank position (see page 62) with your shoulders positioned directly above your wrists. Activate your abdominals and glutes.

- Bend at your elbows to lower your body. Keep your elbows tucked in, close to the side of your ribs.

- At the bottom of the movement, pause and push up through your hands and your feet. Raise your left arm and right leg to a Superman position.

- Bring your arm and leg back down to High Plank position and repeat the move with your other arm and leg to complete the move.

32 | DORSAL RAISES

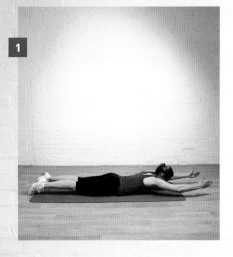

1

HOW TO DO IT:

- Lie face down on the floor with your chin tucked in and eye gaze down. Extend your arms out in front of you in a Superman position.

- Relax your body and, as you inhale, squeeze your glutes and lift your upper torso off the floor.

- Pause at the top of the movement and, with control, lower back down slowly to the starting position to complete the move.

2

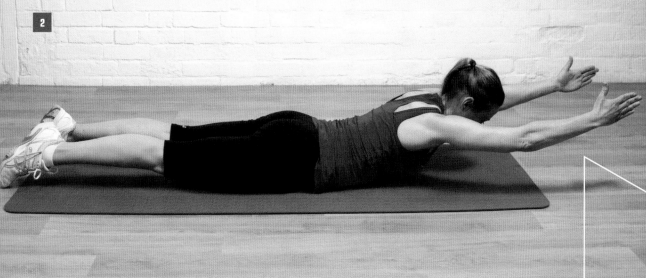

BODYWEIGHT TRAINING

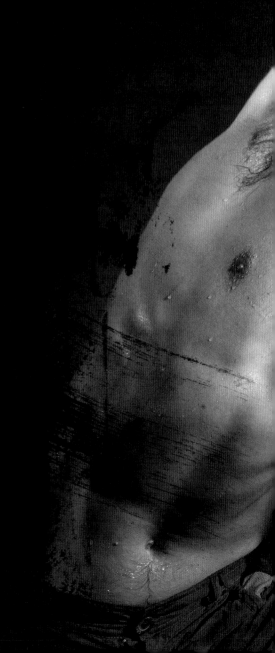

PRIMAL POWER STRETCH

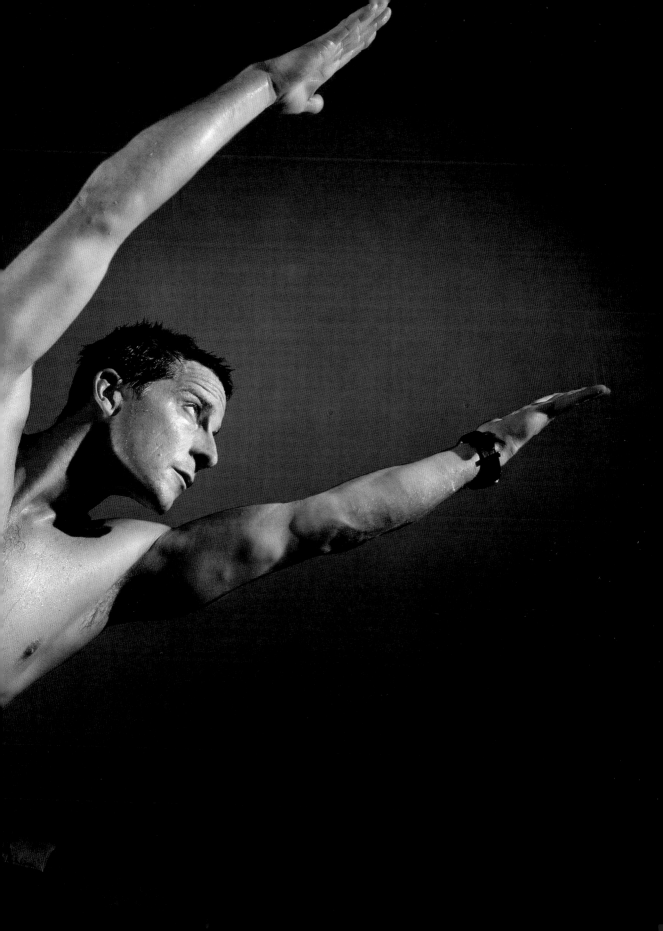

1 | MOUNTAIN POSE

Focus and benefits: improves posture; strengthens mind, thighs, knees, abdominals and glutes.

"

This posture invites you to stand strong and steady – I call it the Everest pose. This is my go-to stance before I begin my Primal Power sequence.

"

HOW TO DO IT:

- Stand tall with your feet together and spread your weight evenly through both feet.

- Inhale, squeeze your kneecaps into your thighs and engage your glutes and abdominals.

- Raise your ribcage and drop your shoulders away from your ears.

- Find focus as you relax your arms at the side of your body and exhale to complete the posture.

2 | EXTENDED MOUNTAIN POSE

Focus and benefits: improves posture; strengthens mind, thighs, knees, abdominals and glutes.

HOW TO DO IT:

- Stand tall with your feet together and spread your weight evenly through both feet.

- Inhale, squeeze your kneecaps into your thighs and engage your glutes and abdominals.

- As you exhale, lift your ribcage away from your hip bones and drop your shoulders away from your ears.

- Inhale and extend your arms overhead, palms facing inwards.

- Keep your shoulders down to create length in the neck as you exhale to complete the posture.

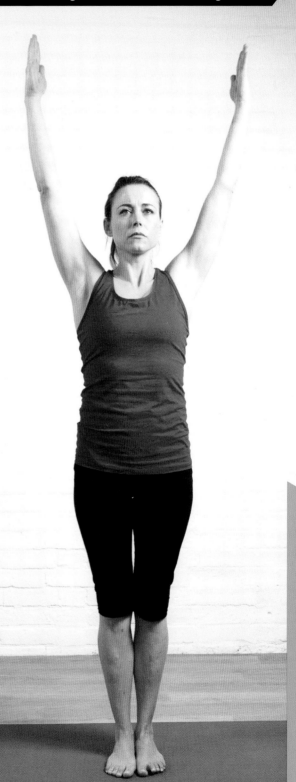

3 | FORWARD FOLD

Focus and benefits: stretches hamstrings and calves; strengthens arms.

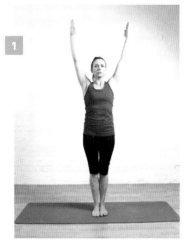

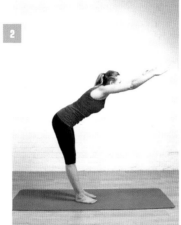

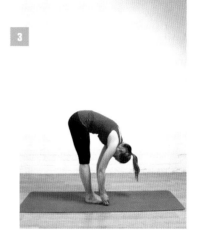

TIP! You may need to keep your knees bent at first, but over time your flexibility will improve. You can make a note of the range of movement in your progress chart (see pages 203–6).

HOW TO DO IT:

- Start in a strong Extended Mountain Pose (see page 103).

- Hinge at your hips, bend your knees and fold forward, keeping your spine as straight as possible.

- Continue to fold until your chest finds your thighs and place your hands on your shins or on the floor.

- As you exhale, slowly straighten your legs and press your palms to the floor on either side of your feet.

- Tuck your chin in to gain a sense of lengthening through your neck to complete the posture.

- Slowly roll up to a standing position to come out of the posture. Be careful to bring your head up last.

4 | PLANK

HOW TO DO IT:

- Lie on the floor facing down, with your shoulders and upper part of your torso propped on your forearms. Your elbows should be aligned beneath your shoulders.

- Lift your bodyweight off the floor, pressing your forearms and toes into the floor and creating a straight line from your head to your feet as you come into Low Plank.

- Keeping a neutral spine alignment, slowly come up on to your wrists into High Plank, bracing through the abdominals and squeezing your kneecaps up towards your thighs.

- Tighten through your glutes and slide your shoulders away from your ears, keeping your eye gaze down towards the floor.

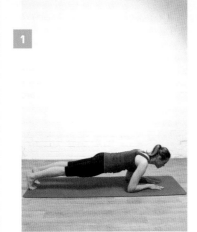

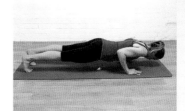

VARIATION:

Stay in Low Plank to help build up your core strength or if you have any wrist problems. Progress to High Plank as your confidence grows and fitness develops.

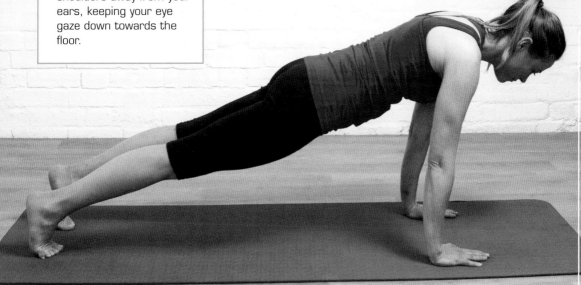

PRIMAL POWER STRETCH

5 | UP DOG

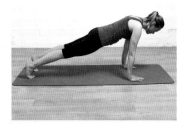

HOW TO DO IT:

■ Start in High Plank position (see page 105). Lower your body towards the floor, keeping your elbows close to your torso. Check your shoulders are aligned directly above your wrists.

■ Continue to lower your body until it makes contact with the floor.

■ Inhale, engage your abdominals and squeeze your glutes to look after your lower back.

■ Straighten your arms to lift your chest away from the floor.

■ As you exhale, draw your shoulders down and away from your ears to create length in your neck.

■ Keep your eye gaze forward and inhale to expand your chest.

■ Exhale and focus on lengthening your spine to complete the movement.

VARIATION:

To advance the move and challenge your body, lift your hips and thighs off the floor and continue to lift your chest in the posture.

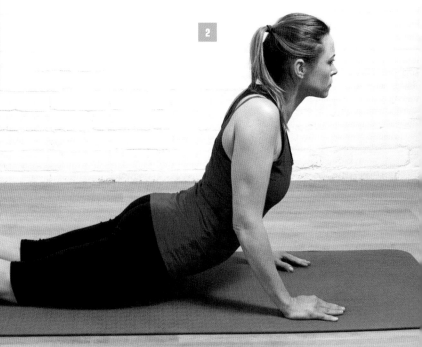

6 | DOWN DOG

Focus and benefits: stretches spine, hamstrings and shoulders; promotes full-body circulation.

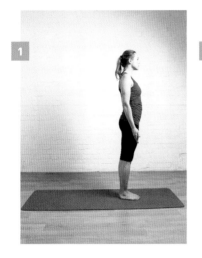
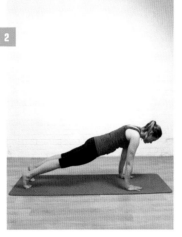
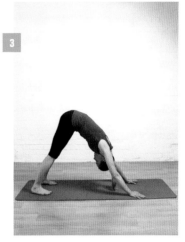

HOW TO DO IT:

- Start in Mountain Pose (see page 102). Fold forwards and reach down to plant the palms of your hands on the floor in front of you. Bend your knees slightly if needed.

- Engage your abdominals and step your feet backwards, one by one, so that you come into High Plank position (see page 105), keeping your palms flat to the floor and your weight forwards.

- Spread your fingers wide for stability and lift your hips towards the ceiling. Keep your knees slightly bent and continue to lift your hips upwards to allow your body to create an inverted V shape.

- Press your heels towards the floor, straighten your legs and deepen the posture by continuing to press your heels into the floor. Keep your arms extended straight.

- Press your chest downwards to straighten your back to enhance the inversion.

TIP! Think 'heavy' head – let the weight of your head hang low – and imagine someone is grabbing you by the belt and lifting your hips up high.

"

This is one of the great yoga stretches for core, back and legs, and I use it a lot when I just need a quick stretch.

"

7 | SPLIT DOWN DOG

Focus and benefits: stretches hamstrings; improves hip flexibility; strengthens arms.

TIP! Aim to keep your standing leg strong and maintain the length in your spine.

HOW TO DO IT:

- Start in Down Dog position (see page 107). Make sure your weight is evenly distributed through your hands during the posture.

- Inhale and, as you exhale, lift your right leg into the air, pressing your heel upwards towards the ceiling. Keep your hips level as you elevate your leg and try not to twist at the hips. Pause.

- Slowly lower your leg back down and rest in your Down Dog position.

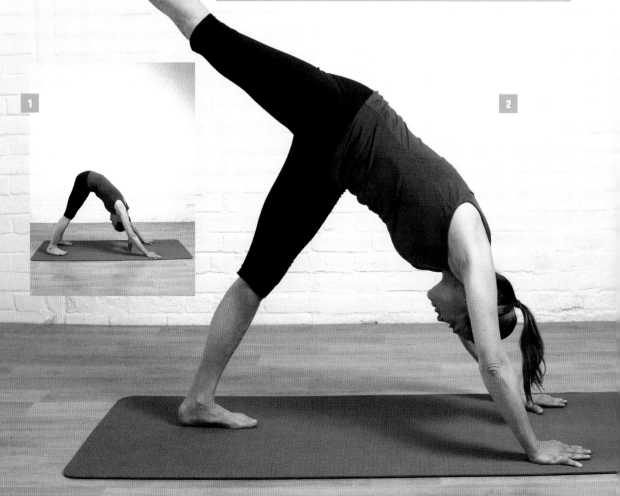

1

2

8 | KNEE PULL-IN

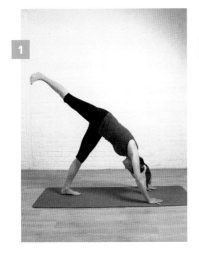
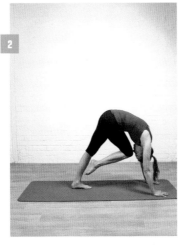
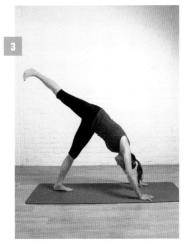

HOW TO DO IT:

- Start in Split Down Dog (see page 108). Make sure your weight is evenly distributed through your hands, your hips are square and your abdominals are activated.

- Bend the knee of your extended leg, bringing it down and in towards your chest. Shift your bodyweight forward to engage your core.

- Extend your upper back forward through your shoulders and continue to bring the knee of your lifted leg into your chest and as close to your nose as possible. Keep your eye gaze down and slightly forwards.

- Extend your leg back to its starting position and re-set to your Split Down Dog position to complete the move.

PRIMAL POWER STRETCH

9 | BOAT POSE

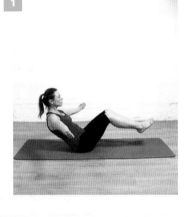

1

HOW TO DO IT:

- Start in a seated position with your knees bent and feet on the floor a hip-width apart.

- Lift your feet off the floor and bring your knees inwards towards your chest.

- Place your hands on the back of your hamstrings to gain balance, if necessary.

- Straighten through your spine and lift your chest. Sit tall from your hips and keep your feet off the floor.

- Lean back under control, until you feel your abdominal brace.

- Focus on your balance and continue to keep your abdominal brace.

- Keeping your feet elevated, begin to extend your legs fully, without compromising your back and chest position, to complete the movement.

2

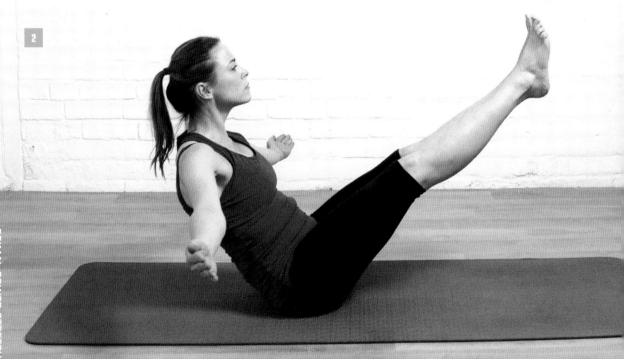

10 | RUSSIAN PRAYER TWIST

Focus and benefits: helps with coordination and balance; strengthens abdominals, hips and thighs.

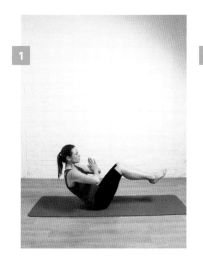
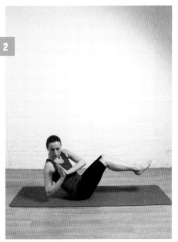
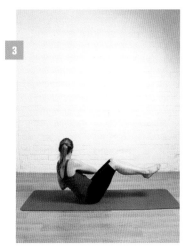

HOW TO DO IT:

- Start in a seated position and straighten through your spine. Sit tall from your hips and keep your knees bent and feet on the floor.

- Lean back under control, until you feel your abdominals tighten.

- Focus on your balance and keep all your core stabilization muscles activated.

- Slowly elevate your feet off the floor and keep your knees bent.

- Press the heels of your hands together into prayer position.

- Slowly twist your upper body to the right, reaching your right elbow behind you.

- Aim to tap your right elbow on the floor behind you, as close to your mid-line as possible.

- Keeping your hips and legs still, twist your upper torso to your left-hand side and tap your left elbow on the floor behind you, again as close to your mid-line as possible.

- Bring your upper body back to a central position, then lower your heels to the floor to complete the move.

11 | STANDING CHAIR

Focus and benefits: strengthens lower body and lower back; stretches shoulders.

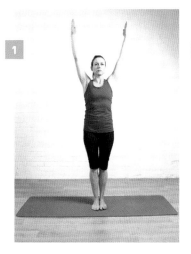

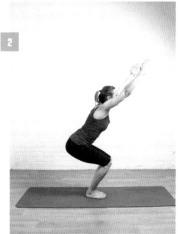

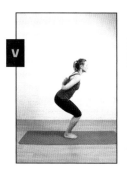

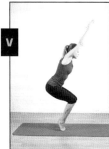

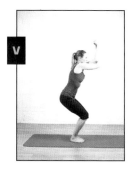

HOW TO DO IT:

- Start in extended Mountain Pose (see page 103). Keep your arms extended above your head and hinge your hips backwards, as if you are about to sit down in a chair. Hold.

- Press your thighs together and lean forward slightly. Draw your shoulders back and down away from your ears, tightening and bracing your abdominals.

- Keep your back straight and eye gaze forward. Turn your hands so your thumbs are pointing upwards and your palms are facing each other.

- Sink deeper into the posture to complete the position.

VARIATIONS:

Prayer hands in front or behind your torso
Draw your shoulders back and press the heels of your hands together into a prayer position. Position them in front of your chest or alternatively behind your back, with your palms positioned between your shoulder blades, fingers pointing upwards.

Standing Chair on your toes
Begin to tip your bodyweight slightly forward as you lift your heels off the floor and come up on to your toes.

Standing Chair, eagle arms
Reach your arms out wide and wrap them together, bringing your left arm under your right, and crossing at the elbows. Cross your arms at your wrists too, and clasp your palms together with your fingertips pointing upwards. Deepen your chair pose and gently pull your arms forwards and away from your upper body to complete the move.

12 | HIP BRIDGE

Focus and benefits: **strengthens abdominals, lower back and legs; opens shoulders and chest; eases anxiety.**

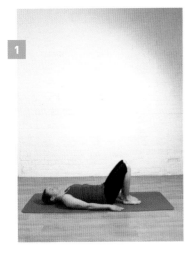

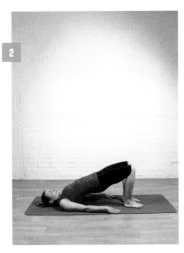

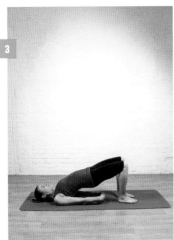

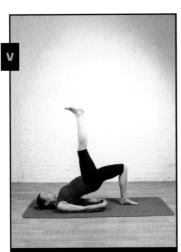

VARIATION:

Single-leg Hip Bridge
Extend and elevate one leg into the air without compromising your spinal alignment.

HOW TO DO IT:

- Lie on your back with your knees bent and feet on the floor a hip-width apart. Rest your arms at your side, palms facing down.

- Press your heels into the ground, squeeze your glutes and lift your hips up off the floor.

- Roll up slowly until your hips are fully extended. Keep the top of your shoulders in contact with the floor.

- Clasp your hands together under your hips. To advance the move, tuck your shoulders under to open further through your chest to complete the posture.

13 | WARRIOR ONE

Focus and benefits: strengthens lower body; tones abdominals; opens hips.

HOW TO DO IT:

- Start in extended Mountain Pose (see page 103). Step your right foot back behind you approximately twice hip-width.

- Drop your shoulders and brace your abdominals.

- Turn your right foot outwards at 45 degrees.

- Bend your left knee and drop down into a low lunge position. Make sure your knee is directly stacked above your ankle.

- Turn your right hip forwards to bring your hips in a line and keep them square to your shoulders.

- Lean forwards slightly from your waist, maintaining a straight back.

- Lift your ribcage away from your hips and extend your arms upwards, palms facing inwards and thumbs to the ceiling.

- Inhale, lift your chest and press your shoulders back, bringing your eye gaze towards your hands, to complete the position.

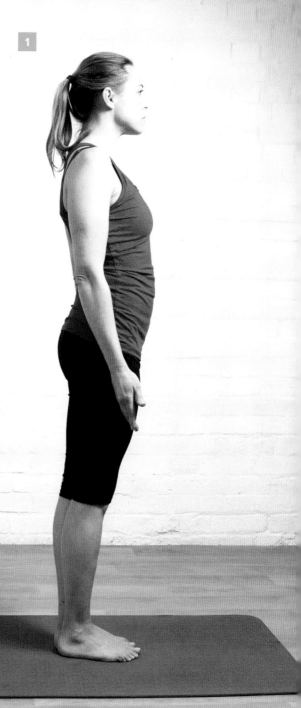

1

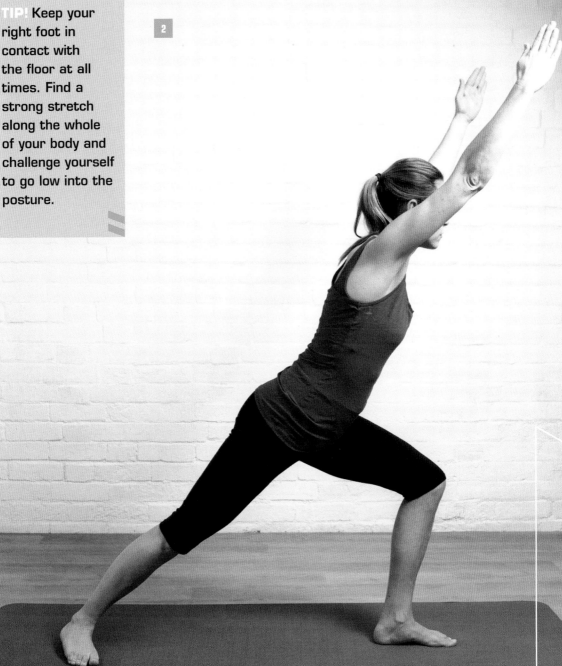

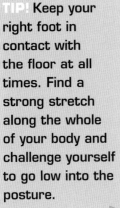

TIP! Keep your right foot in contact with the floor at all times. Find a strong stretch along the whole of your body and challenge yourself to go low into the posture.

Focus and benefits: improves postural awareness and hip flexibility; strengthens lower body.

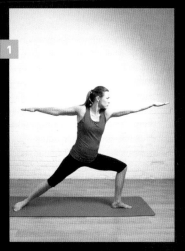

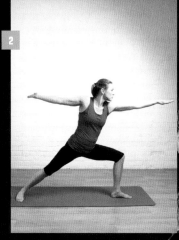

HOW TO DO IT:

- Stand with your feet approximately twice hip-width apart, spread your hands over your ribs and as you inhale allow your ribs to lift away from your hip bones to create space.

- Turn your left foot out at approximately 90 degrees and turn your right foot slightly inwards at 45 degrees.

- Bend your left knee and check it is positioned directly over your ankle.

- Fully extend your arms out to your sides so that they are parallel to the floor. Turn your head towards your left shoulder.

- Turn your left palm down and your right palm up towards the ceiling. Stretch from fingertip to fingertip to open across your chest and energize your whole body.

- Inhale and, as you exhale, settle deeper into the pose, with your eye gaze along the middle and index fingers of your right hand.

- Drop your shoulders away from your ears to lengthen the neck and complete the posture.

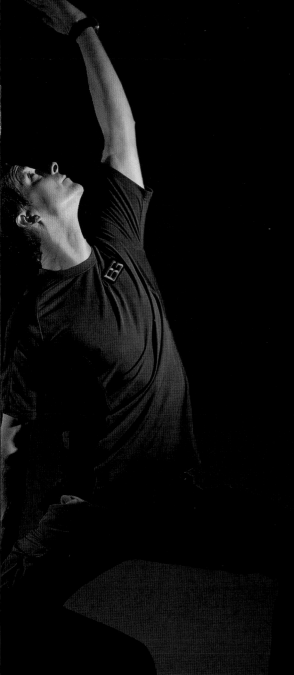

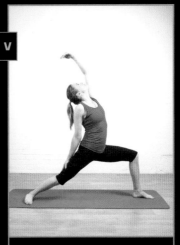

VARIATION:

Reverse Warrior Two

- From Warrior Two position, slowly lift your left arm towards the ceiling and lean backwards from the waist, keeping your left knee and right leg in position.

- Turn your left hand so that your palm faces towards your face.

- Drop your right thigh and continue to look up as you extend your left arm backwards.

- Keep your eye gaze upwards towards the palm of your left hand.

- Continue to lean until you feel a stretch in your side.

15 | WARRIOR LUNGE AND REACH

Focus and benefits: strengthens lower legs and glutes; improves balance; promotes a strong alignment through the body.

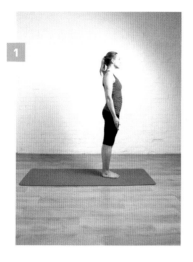

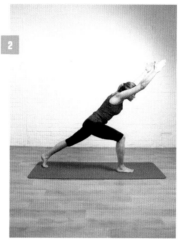

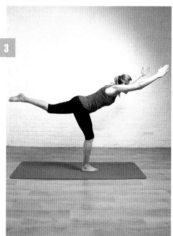

TIP! If the full expression of the posture is a little challenging to begin with, build up to it by hinging forward only part of the way. Keep your upper torso and elevated leg in a straight line and touch your toes back to the floor if you need to regain your balance.

HOW TO DO IT:

- Start in Mountain Pose (see page 102). Take a big step back with your left leg to create strong split lunge position with your feet a hip-width apart, or slightly wider for more balance.

- Extend your arms over your head and brace your abdominals. Transfer your weight on to your right leg and gently lift your left foot off the floor into a single-leg stance, keeping your hips forward and square.

- Focus and find your balance. Hinge forward at the waist and lower your body until your left leg, torso and arms are parallel to the floor, eye gaze down.

- Maintain a strong, straight line from your shoulders to your feet, keeping your neck in line with your spine.

- Keep the hips parallel to the floor as you hold steady to complete the posture.

- As you exhale, release back into the lunge position and then slowly bring your left foot in to meet your right and return to Mountain Pose.

16 | TRIANGLE

Focus and benefits: full body stretch; strengthens thighs, knees and ankles; mobilizes back and stretches oblique abdominals.

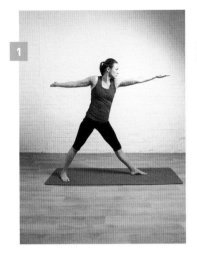

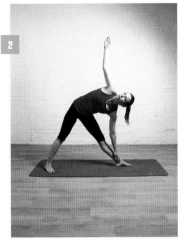

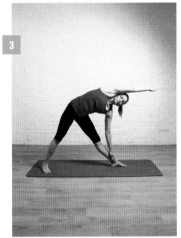

HOW TO DO IT:

- Stand with your feet twice hip-width apart, with your hips parallel to your shoulders.

- Turn your right foot inwards 45 degrees. Turn your left foot outwards 90 degrees.

- Stretch your arms out sideways from your body at shoulder height so that they are perpendicular to the floor and you create a T-shape with your body, palms facing upwards.

- Push your hips backwards towards your right foot and straighten your left leg.

- Squeeze your left knee up tight into your thigh.

- Move your eye gaze to your right hand, slowly windmill your upper body towards your left leg, resting your left hand on your left shin.

- Extend your right arm into the air and pull your right shoulder back. Open your hips by pushing them forwards to complete the posture.

TIP! Imagine you are sandwiched between two panes of glass. Aim for perfect, whole-body alignment.

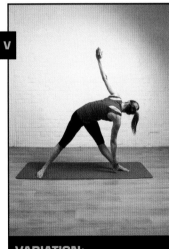

VARIATION:

Triangle Twist
Rotate your upper body 180 degrees to create a closed twist triangle.

17 | TREE POSE

Focus and benefits: improves balance; strengthens core, lower body and spine.

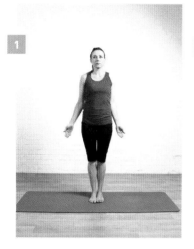
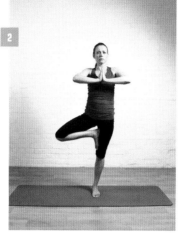
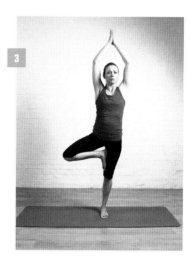

TIP! Your lifted knee should be at 90 degrees to your hip. If balance is an issue, keep your lifted leg close to the floor or touching the ankle of your supporting ankle.

HOW TO DO IT:

- Start in Mountain Pose (see page 102). Inhale, engage your abdominal muscles, find your focus and balance as you exhale.

- Slowly lift your right leg and place the ball and heel of your right foot on the inside of your supporting left leg.

- With your chest lifted and your hips square and open, draw your shoulders back and press the heels of your hands together into prayer position, keeping them close to your chest. Squeeze the knee of your supporting leg into the thigh muscle.

- Extend your arms over your head in prayer position and hold to complete the movement.

- To come back to starting point, lower your arms and your leg down to Mountain Pose.

18 | EAGLE POSE

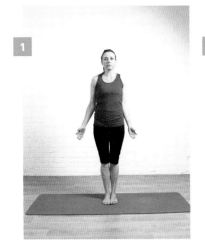

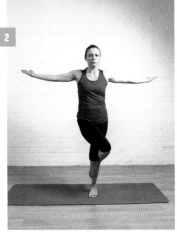

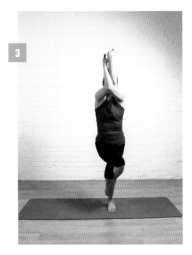

HOW TO DO IT:

- Start in Mountain Pose (see page 102). Find your focus and balance.

- Lift your right leg off the floor and wrap it up and over your supporting left leg. Hook your right foot behind your left calf to create a single-leg stance.

- Reach your arms out wide and then wrap them together, bringing your left arm under your right, and crossing at the elbows.

- Cross your arms at your wrists too, and clasp your palms together. Aim to point your fingertips upwards towards the ceiling.

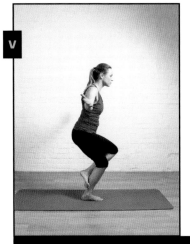

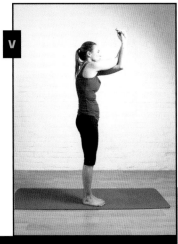

VARIATION:

Break the posture down into eagle legs or arms only. The deeper you go the harder it gets!

- Sink deeper into your single-leg stance and bring your elbows up to chin height.

- Straighten upwards from the hips and gently pull your arms forwards and away from your body to create a stretch through your upper back to complete the movement.

PRIMAL POWER STRETCH

19 | CROW POSE

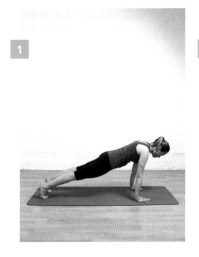

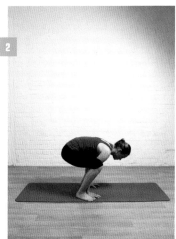

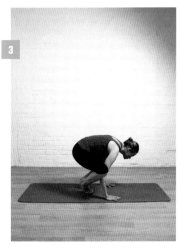

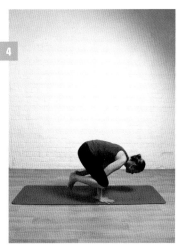

HOW TO DO IT:

- Start in High Plank position (see page 105). Walk, step or jump both feet forwards towards your hands. Your feet should land at the outside of your hands.

- Keep your hips low, engage your abdominals and bend your elbows so they are ready to support your body weight.

- Gently press your bent elbows into the insides of your knees.

- Walk your feet together so that your big toes are touching.

- Keep your eye gaze forward and focus to get ready to take the challenge.

- Lift your toes off the floor and keep your body tucked in tight as you lean forwards and balance your weight on your arms.

PRIMAL POWER STRETCH

> "
> This posture is one of my key fundamentals and I love the challenge of the arm balance as well as the focused mindset it requires. It's a great move to master and it's one posture that really stretches out my upper back. However, be warned . . . it can take a while to perfect. Just keep trying – it will come!
> "

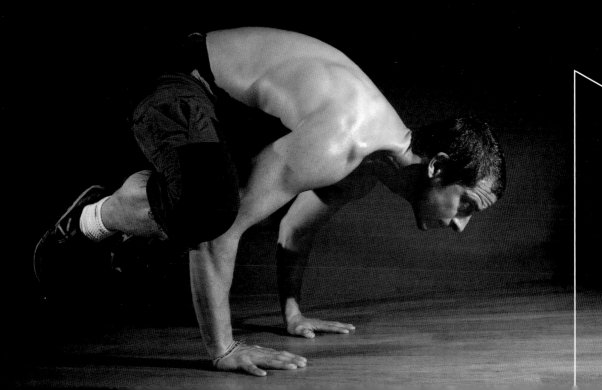

20 | SIDE STAND TO T STAND

Focus and benefits: stretches shoulders, chest, arms and core; focuses on balance and core strength.

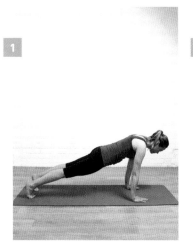
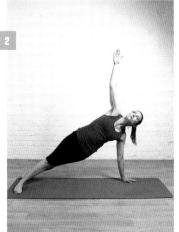
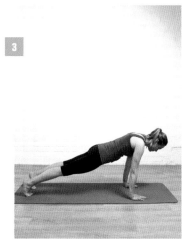

HOW TO DO IT:

- Start in High Plank position (see page 105) and walk your feet out to a shoulder-width apart.

- Make sure your hands are positioned directly under your shoulders. Maintain a straight line from your toes to your shoulders.

- Tighten through your abdominals, then lift your right arm off the floor and point your arm upwards towards the ceiling, simultaneously rotating your hips and feet to one side. The hips should be stacked.

- Hold this position with a straight line from your shoulders to your ankles, with your arm extended overhead.

- Lower your arm and rotate your hips and feet back to High Plank position. Pause.

- Re-adjust to make sure your weight is forward and your abdominals, glutes and thighs are activated.

- Repeat the rotation on the other side to complete the movement.

PRIMAL POWER STRETCH

21 | EXTENDED BEAR POSE

Focus and benefits: stretches lower back and arms; helps relaxation.

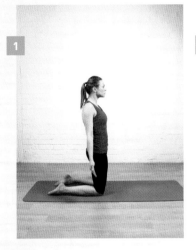

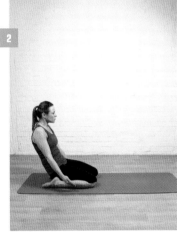

HOW TO DO IT:

- Bring yourself into an upright kneeling position, arms at your sides.

- Spread your knees a shoulder-width apart and sit back on to your heels.

- Hinge forwards from your hips and fold your upper body forwards to bring your forehead to the floor.

- Extend your arms forwards and, within your own range of movement, bring your chest to your knees.

- Use your breath to surrender to the pose, lowering your chest as far as possible, and relax to complete the movement.

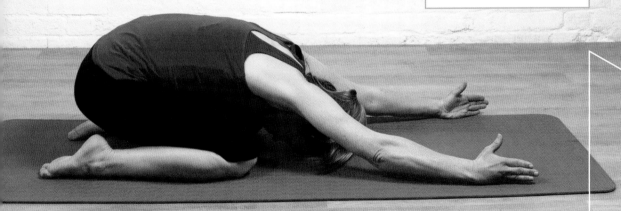

22 | WILD THING

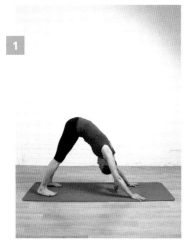

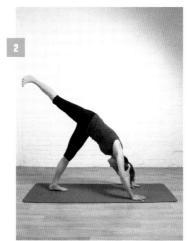

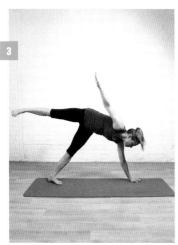

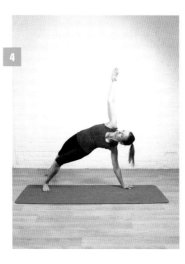

HOW TO DO IT:

- Begin in Down Dog position (see page 107).

- Lift your right leg into the air and press your heel towards the ceiling.

- Bend your right knee and bring your heel towards your buttocks, allowing your hips and body to rotate slightly.

- Begin to transfer your bodyweight on to your left arm and the outer part of your left foot.

- Lift your right arm off the floor and continue to rotate your body towards the ceiling. Allow your eye gaze to follow your arm.

- Drop your right foot to the floor and squeeze your glutes to lift your hips to the ceiling to mimic a backbend.

- Press your toes into the floor and lift your heels. If it feels comfortable, allow your head to drop back and extend your right arm.

- To complete the pose, drop your hips towards the floor and reverse the move slowly to find your way back to Down Dog.

- Repeat the movement on the other side of the body.

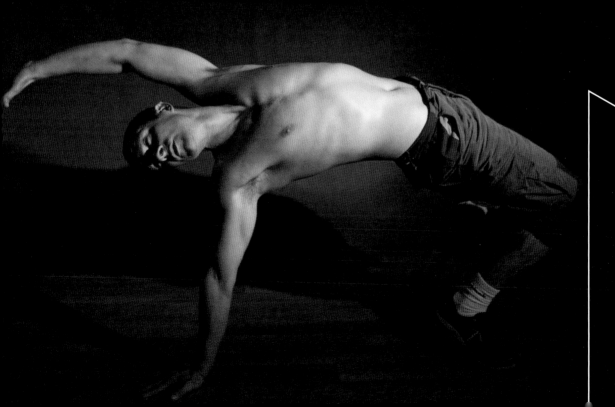

"

If ever there was an exercise to make you feel like a beast this is it – essentially inspired by a love of scaling rockfaces and having to negotiate precarious positions! Often I am gripping on with the balls of my feet, toes curled tight, arching backwards to gain just a little extra traction with my hand.

Adding this Hero move into your workouts is always fun . . . oh, and it keeps me strong and supple for those back flips I taught myself when I turned 30 years old!

"

PRIMAL POWER STRETCH

5 | THE WORKOUTS

'Train insane or remain the same.'

There is no easy way and there are no shortcuts to getting fit and staying fit. It takes good old honest hard work, sweat and motivation to be in the best shape of your life. Commitment is the key to success, as you have seen reinforced and reiterated throughout this book – so let's get going and work out!

BEFORE YOU WORK OUT, WARM UP

Before you train hard, warm up properly. This is vital. Trust me, it will improve your performance and reduce your chances of injury. The warm-up for me has become more than just preparation for intensive exercise. I have realized that by entering a warm-up sequence it helps prepare me mentally for the workout ahead.

These dynamic warm-ups are made up of continuous, whole-body movement sequences and aim to coordinate all your moving parts (ligaments, joints, muscles) by challenging your range of motion, strength and balance all in one. They aim to:

■ improve movement patterns
■ improve coordination
■ increase mobility in your joints
■ raise muscle temperature

■ increase blood flow to your muscles
■ prepare your nervous system (nerve-to-muscle pathways) for the increased activity
■ improve performance
■ reduce risk of injury

A good, effective warm-up will mimic the movements of your main workout. With this in mind, I have included a dynamic warm-up sequence specific to each discipline: Kettlebell, Bodyweight and Primal Power Stretch, plus a mixed-discipline warm-up for the Hero workouts.

Remember: the warm-up should start slow and progress quickly.

The warm-ups can feel like a mini-workout in themselves. That's OK – it's in the plan and they are a great way to start your training.

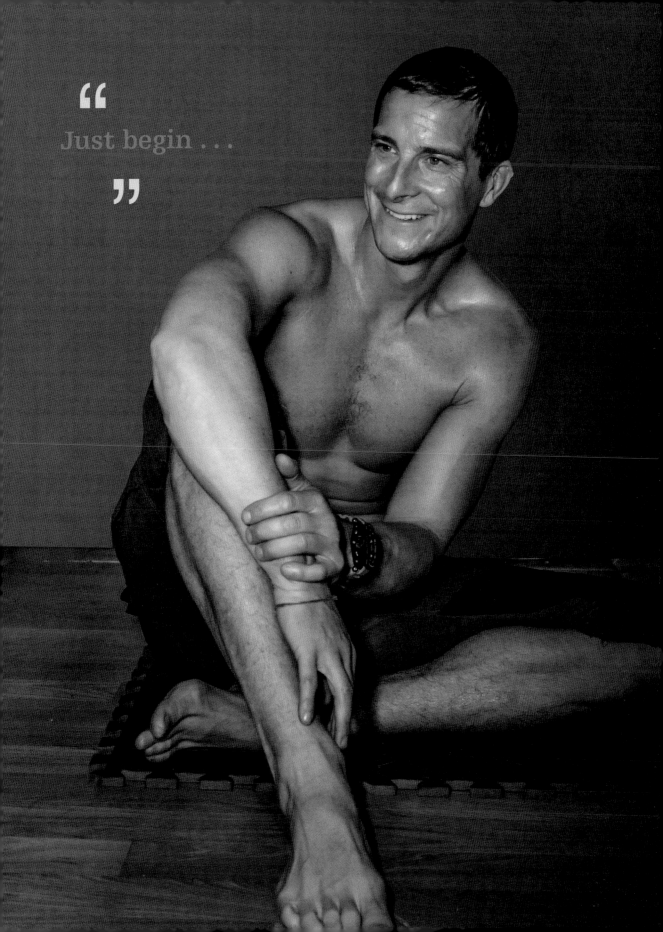

"

Just begin . . .

"

KETTLEBELL WARM-UP

x8

Shoulder Rolls, forwards
and backwards

x8

Arm Circles, forwards
and backwards

x8

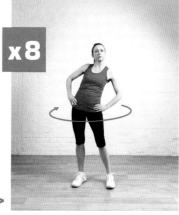

Hip Circles, right

x8

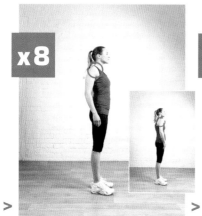

Hip Circles, left

x8

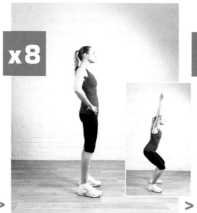

Hip Drives

x8

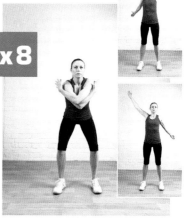

Squat with Hug and
Diagonal Open

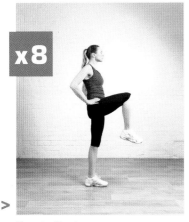

Knee to Chest

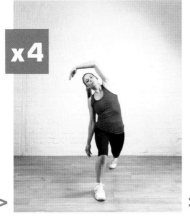

Lunges with side bend, right

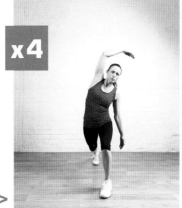

Lunges with side bend, left

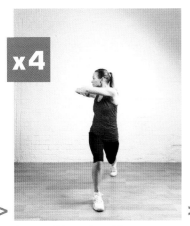

Lunges with rotation, right

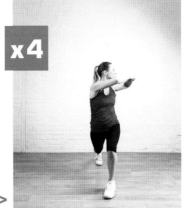

Lunges with rotation, left

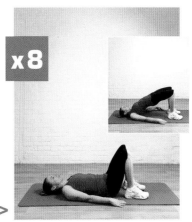

Hip Bridge Dips (see page 85)

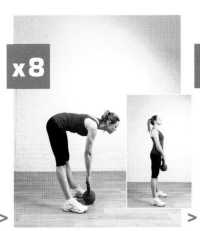

Kettlebell Deadlifts (see page 34)

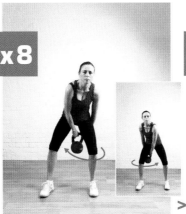

Standing Abdominal 8s (see page 32)

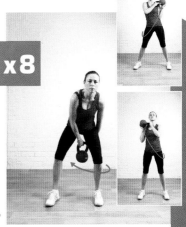

Alternating Abdominal 8s
to Woodchops (see page 33)

BODYWEIGHT WARM-UP

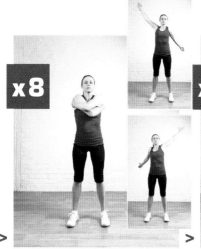

x8

Shoulder Rolls,
forwards and backwards

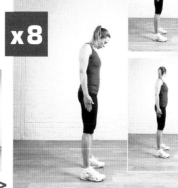

x8

Head Drop and Turns

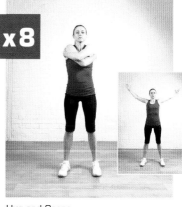

x8

Hug and Opens

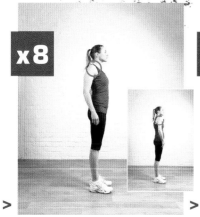

x8

Hug and Diagonal Opens

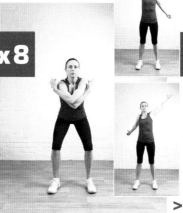

x8

Squat with Hug and
Diagonal Open

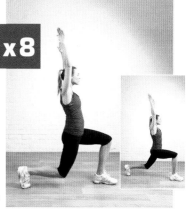

x8

Alternating Lunges, forwards

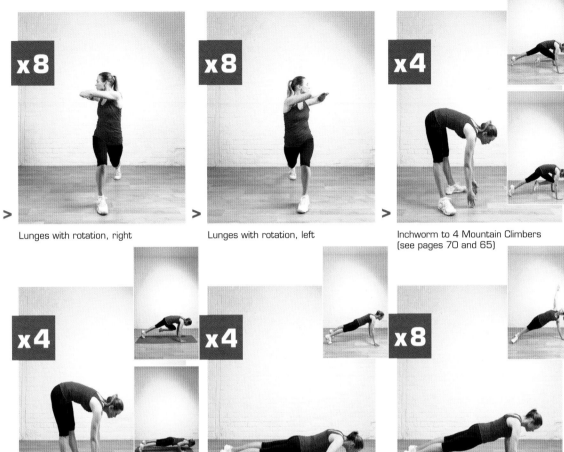

> Lunges with rotation, right

> Lunges with rotation, left

> Inchworm to 4 Mountain Climbers (see pages 70 and 65)

> Inchworm to 4 Cross Mountain Climbers with a Push-up (see pages 70 and 66)

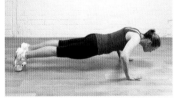

> Push-ups into Primal Push-ups

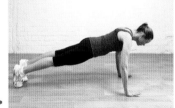

> T Push-up

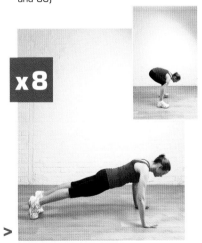

> Bear Leap and Reach (see page 67)

PRIMAL POWER STRETCH WARM-UP

POSTURE CHECK AND FINDING **NEUTRAL SPINE POSITION** (see page 25).

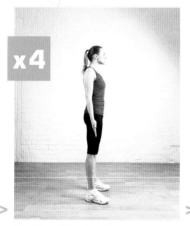

Breaths in Mountain Pose
(see page 102)

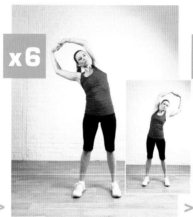

Standing Side Stretches

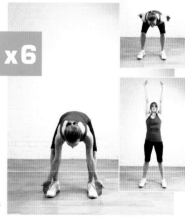

Sweep the Floor and Rises

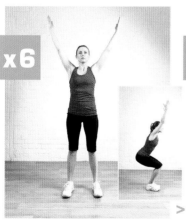

Extended Mountain Pose to
Standing Chair (see pages 103 and 112)

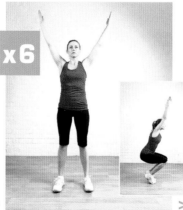

Extended Mountain Pose to
Standing Chair, on toes

x6

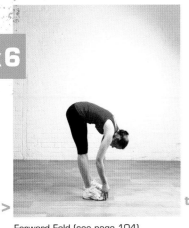

Forward Fold (see page 104)

to

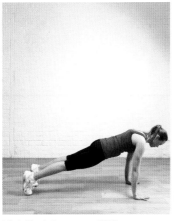

High Plank (see page 105)

to

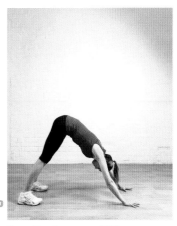

Down Dog (see page 107)

to

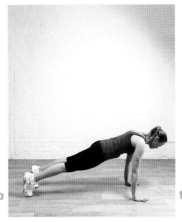

High Plank

to

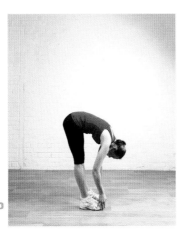

Forward Fold

If your workout doesn't challenge you, it won't change you.

HERO WARM-UP

x4

Head Turns, right

x4

Head Turns, left

x8

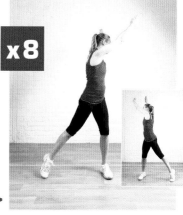

Torso Twists, with reach

x8

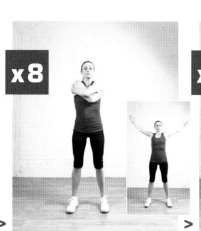

Hug and Opens

x8

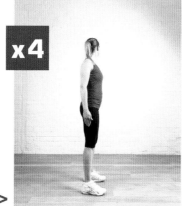

Hug and Diagonal Opens

x8

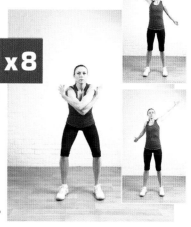

Squat with Hug and
Diagonal Opens

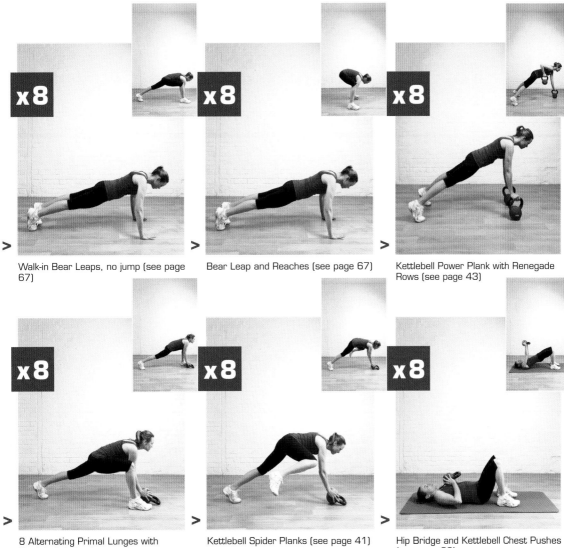

x8

> Walk-in Bear Leaps, no jump (see page 67)

x8

> Bear Leap and Reaches (see page 67)

x8

> Kettlebell Power Plank with Renegade Rows (see page 43)

x8

> 8 Alternating Primal Lunges with Kettlebell, ball grip

x8

> Kettlebell Spider Planks (see page 41)

x8

> Hip Bridge and Kettlebell Chest Pushes (see page 36)

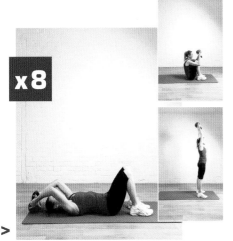

x8

> Kettlebell Abdominal Crunch to Standings (see page 39)

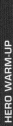

BEAR'S COOL DOWNS

Once you have completed your workout, cool down.

The cool down part of your workouts allows your body to recover after intensive exercise. Again, don't skip them – they are a vital part of your training. I use my cool down to bring my breathing, body temperature and heart rate back down to normal, and to make it super-effective I like to add in a total body stretch.

To cool down I complete a short routine of exercises similar to my warm-ups but with no weights and less intensity, followed by a stretch sequence. Hold each of the stretches for 20+ seconds. As the feeling of the stretch wears off, deepen the stretch again to increase the flexibility of the muscles you are stretching.

COOL-DOWN ROUTINE

Slowly bring your heart rate down by completing the following exercises at low intensity:

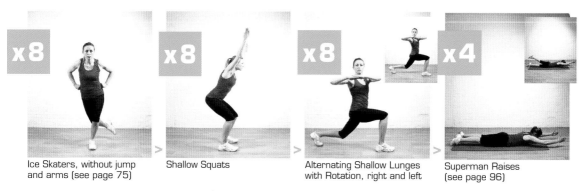

Ice Skaters, without jump and arms (see page 75)

Shallow Squats

Alternating Shallow Lunges with Rotation, right and left

Superman Raises (see page 96)

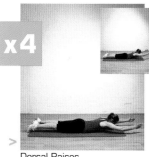

Dorsal Raises (see page 99)

STRETCH SEQUENCE

Hold each stretch for 30–45 seconds.

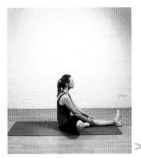

Hamstring Stretch,
right and left

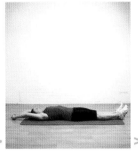

Floor Abdominal Stretch

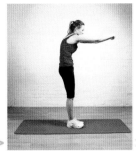

Upper Back Stretch

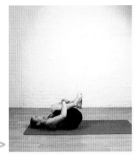

Lower Back Stretch

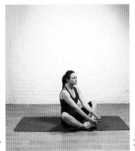

Adductor Stretch

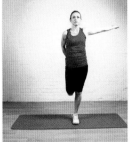

Quad Stretch,
right and left

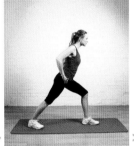

Calf Stretch,
right and left

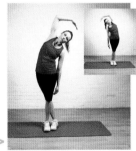

Oblique Stretch,
right and left

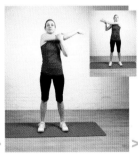

Shoulder Stretch,
right and left

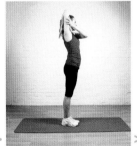

Tricep Stretch,
right and left

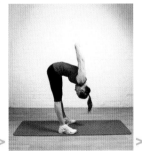

Combined Shoulder and
Hamstring Stretch

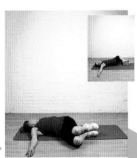

Spine Rotation Stretch,
right and left

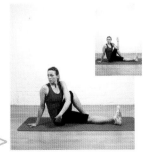

Seated Twist,
right and left

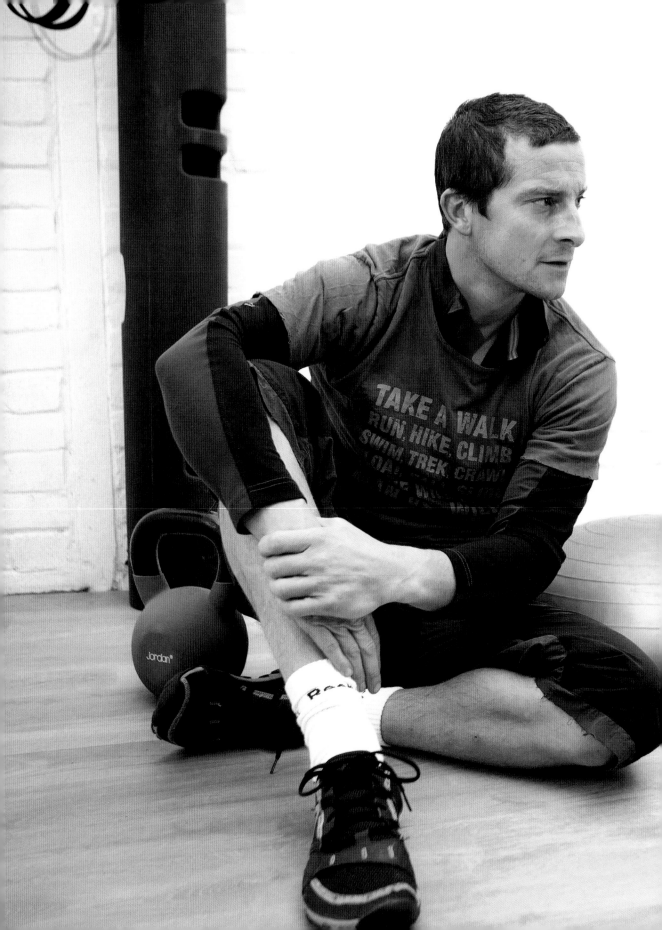

FOCUSED WORKOUTS

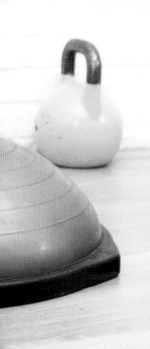

OK, are we ready to hit the workouts? The following focused workouts have been designed to help improve your fitness, make you stronger, reduce your body fat and increase your lean muscle mass.

They are divided up by training discipline (Kettlebell, Bodyweight and Primal Power Stretch) and body part (lower body, upper body and whole body). In addition, I have shared with you my focused Hero workouts. These are tough workouts designed to accelerate your training, break the routine and keep shocking your muscles! Aim to throw one of them into your training schedules once a week.

KETTLEBELL WORKOUT ONE

WHOLE BODY TIME: **10 MINUTES, 20 MINUTES OR 30 MINUTES**

COMPLETE THE FOLLOWING BLOCKS OF EXERCISES ONCE FOR AN APPROXIMATELY 10-MINUTE WORKOUT;
TWICE FOR A 20-MINUTE WORKOUT; OR THREE TIMES FOR A 30-MINUTE WORKOUT.

EQUIPMENT: KETTLEBELLS, MAT

COMPLETE YOUR **KETTLEBELL WARM-UP** (see pages 130–1).

BLOCK ONE | Complete the following sequence of exercises to make one round.
Complete as many rounds as possible in 4 minutes.

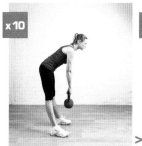 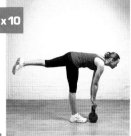 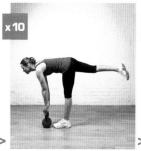 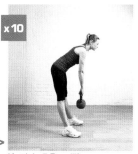

Kettlebell Deadlifts (see page 34) > Single-leg Deadlifts, left (see page 35) > Single-leg Deadlifts, right > Kettlebell Deadlifts

REST FOR 1 MINUTE

BLOCK TWO | Complete the following sequence of exercises.
Work for 20 seconds and rest for 10 seconds between exercises.

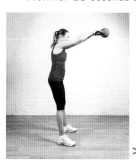 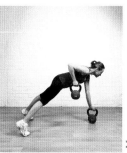 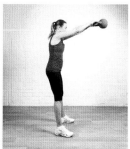 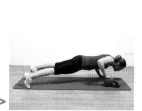

Double-hand Swing (see page 31) > Kettlebell Power Plank with Renegade Row (see page 43) > Double-hand Swing > Kettlebell Power Push-ups (see page 53)

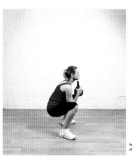 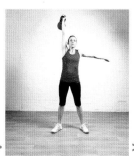 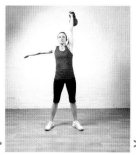 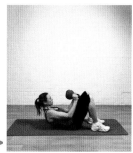

Goblet Squats (see page 45) > Kettlebell Front Squat to Press, right (see page 44) > Kettlebell Front Squat to Press, left > Abdominal Pull-in (see page 38)

REST FOR 1 MINUTE

RECOVER AND COMPLETE A **FULL-BODY COOL DOWN** (see pages 138–9).

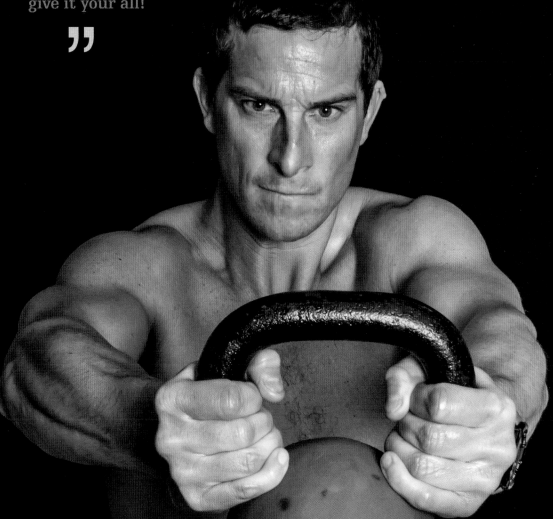

"

Before you embark on these epic Kettlebell workouts,
I have a last piece of advice – one that you will often
hear being called out during my training sessions with
Natalie and one that certainly echoes in my head when
I'm about to train solo in some jungle or on our island:

Cuidado! Cast-iron objects overhead can cause serious
injury. Respect the kettlebell . . . Now get started and
give it your all!

"

KETTLEBELL WORKOUT TWO
WHOLE BODY; EMPHASIS UPPER BODY

TIME: 30 MINUTES

EQUIPMENT: KETTLEBELLS, MAT

COMPLETE YOUR **KETTLEBELL WARM-UP** (see pages 130–1).

BLOCK ONE | Complete the following sequence of exercises.
Work for 20 seconds and rest for 10 seconds between exercises.

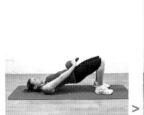 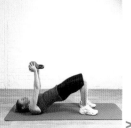 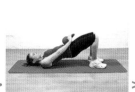 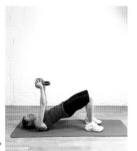

Hip Bridge Pull-in (see page 37) > Hip Bridge and Kettlebell Chest Push (see page 36) > Hip Bridge Pull-in > Hip Bridge and Kettlebell Chest Push

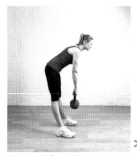 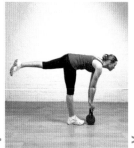 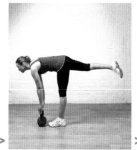 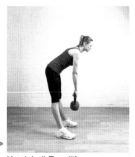

Kettlebell Deadlift (see page 34) > Single-leg Deadlift, left (see page 35) > Single-leg Deadlift, right > Kettlebell Deadlift

REST FOR 30 SECONDS

BLOCK TWO | Complete the following sequence of exercises.
Work for 20 seconds and rest for 10 seconds between exercises.

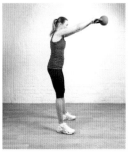 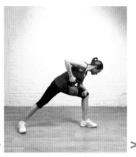 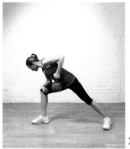 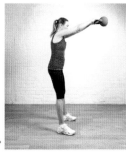

Double-hand Swing (see page 31) > One-arm Kettlebell Row (Warrior Legs), right (see page 40) > One-arm Kettlebell Row (Warrior Legs), left > Double-hand Swing

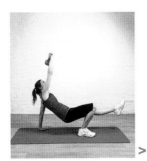
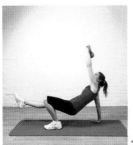
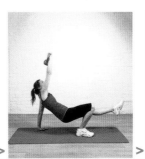
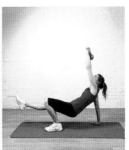

Turkish Get-up Half, right (see page 57) > Turkish Get-up Half, left > Turkish Get-up Half, right > Turkish Get-up Half, left

REST FOR 30 SECONDS

BLOCK THREE | Complete the following sequence of exercises. Work for 20 seconds and rest for 10 seconds between exercises.

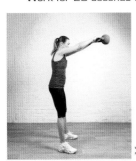
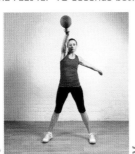
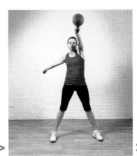
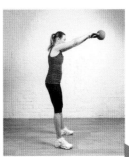

Double-hand Swing (see page 31) > Single-hand Swing, right (see page 30) > Single-hand Swing, left > Double-hand Swing

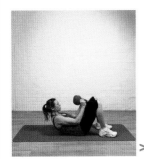
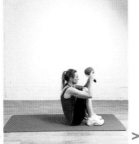
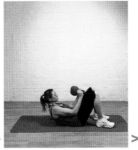
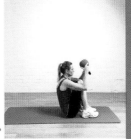

Abdominal Pull-in (see page 38) > Abdominal Crunch to Standing (see page 39) > Abdominal Pull-in > Abdominal Crunch to Standing

REST FOR 30 SECONDS

CONTINUES OVERLEAF

CONTINUED FROM PAGE 145

BLOCK FOUR | Complete the following sequence of exercises. Work for 20 seconds and rest for 10 seconds between exercises.

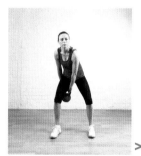

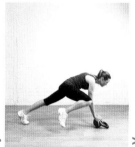

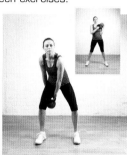

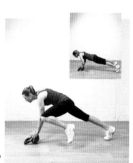

Standing Abdominal 8s (see page 32)

Kettlebell Spider Plank, right and left (see page 41)

Standing Abdominal 8s to Woodchop (see page 33)

Kettlebell Spider Plank and Diamond Push-up (see pages 41 and 52)

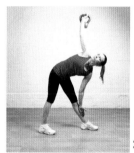

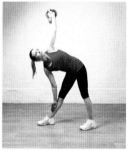

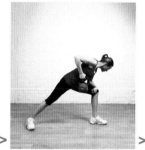

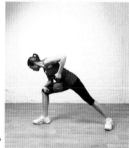

Kettlebell Windmill, right (see page 51)

Kettlebell Windmill, left

One-arm Kettlebell Row (Warrior Legs), right (see page 40)

One-arm Kettlebell Row (Warrior Legs), left

REST FOR 30 SECONDS

BLOCK FIVE | Complete the following sequence of exercises. Work for 20 seconds and rest for 10 seconds between exercises.

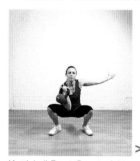

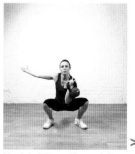

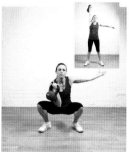

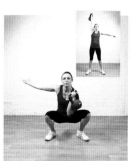

Kettlebell Front Squat, right (see page 44)

Kettlebell Front Squat, left

Kettlebell Front Squat to Press, right (see page 44)

Kettlebell Front Squat to Press, left

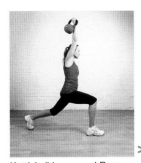

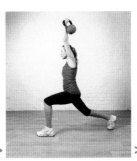

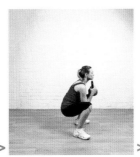

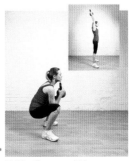

Kettlebell Lunge and Press, right (see page 48)

>

Kettlebell Lunge and Press, left

>

Goblet Squat (see page 45)

>

Goblet Squat and Press (see page 45)

REST FOR 30 SECONDS

BLOCK SIX | Complete the following sequence of exercises back to back with no rest to make one round. Complete as many rounds as possible in 3 minutes.

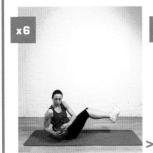

x6

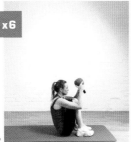

x6

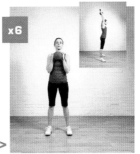

x6

Kettlebell Russian Twists (see pages 54–5)

>

Abdominal Crunches to Standing (see page 39)

>

Bicep to Double-hand Military Presses (see page 49)

REST FOR 1 MINUTE

RECOVER AND COMPLETE A **FULL-BODY COOL DOWN** (see pages 138–9).

KETTLEBELL WORKOUT THREE
WHOLE BODY; EMPHASIS UPPER BODY AND CORE

TIME: 30 MINUTES

EQUIPMENT: KETTLEBELLS, MAT

COMPLETE YOUR **KETTLEBELL WARM-UP** (see pages 130–1).

BLOCK ONE | Complete the following sequence of exercises back to back with no rest to make one round. Complete as many rounds as possible in 6 minutes.

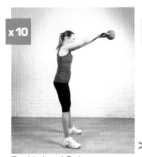

Double-hand Swings (see page 31)

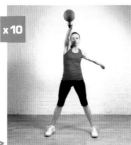

Single-hand Swings, right (see page 30)

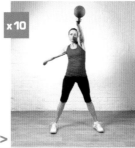

Single-hand Swings, left

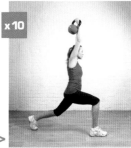

Kettlebell Lunge and Press, right (see page 48)

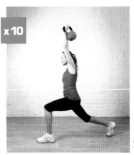

Kettlebell Lunge and Press, left

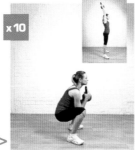

Goblet Squat and Press (see page 45)

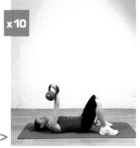

Kettlebell Chest Press (see page 50)

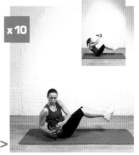

Bear Twist and Press (see page 55)

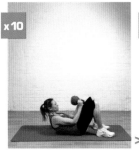

Abdominal Pull-ins (see page 38)

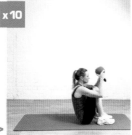

Abdominal Crunch to Standing (see page 39)

REST FOR 1 MINUTE

BLOCK TWO | Complete the following sequence of exercises. Work for 20 seconds and rest for 10 seconds between exercises.

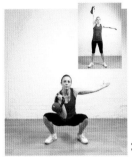

Kettlebell Front Squat to Press, right (see page 44)

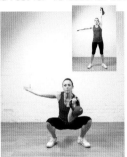

Kettlebell Front Squat to Press, left

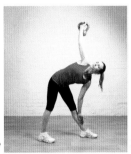

Kettlebell Windmill, right (see page 51)

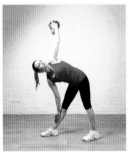

Kettlebell Windmill, left

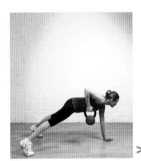

Kettlebell Power Plank with Row, right (see page 42)

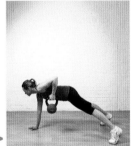

Kettlebell Power Plank with Row, left

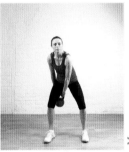

Kettlebell Standing Abdominal 8s (see page 32)

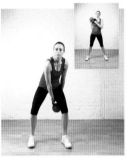

Kettlebell Standing Abdominal 8s to Woodchop (see page 33)

REST FOR 1 MINUTE

BLOCK THREE | Complete each of the following exercises for one minute, performing them back to back.

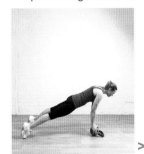

Kettlebell Power Plank, ball grip (see page 41)

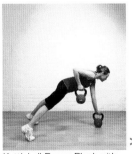

Kettlebell Power Plank with Renegade Row (see page 43)

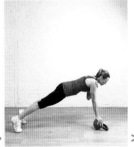

Kettlebell Single-arm Plank, right (see page 41)

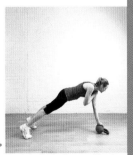

Kettlebell Single-arm Plank, left

REST FOR 30 SECONDS

CONTINUES OVERLEAF

BEAR'S KETTLEBELL WORKOUTS

KETTLEBELL WORKOUT THREE

CONTINUED FROM PAGE 149

BLOCK FOUR | Complete each of the following exercises for 20 seconds and rest for 10 seconds between exercises.

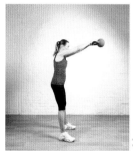 > 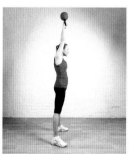 > 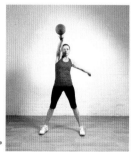 >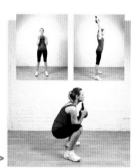

Double-hand Swing (see page 31)

Overhead Swing (see page 31)

Alternating Single-hand Swing, right and left (see page 30)

Goblet Squat to Bicep to Double-hand Military Press (see pages 45 and 49)

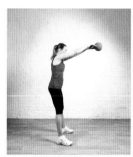 > 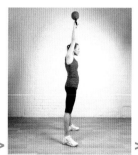 > 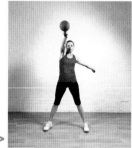 >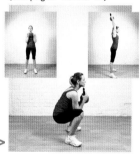

Double-hand Swing

Overhead Swing

Alternating Single-hand Swing, right and left

Goblet Squat to Bicep to Double-hand Military Press

REST FOR 30 SECONDS

BLOCK FIVE | Complete the following sequence of exercises back to back with no rest to make one round. Complete as many rounds as possible in 4 minutes.

x5 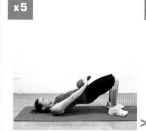 > x5 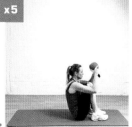 > x5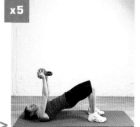

Hip Bridge Pull-ins (see page 37)

Abdominal Crunch to Standing (see page 39)

Hip Bridge and Kettlebell Chest Pushes (see page 36)

REST FOR 1 MINUTE

RECOVER AND COMPLETE A **FULL-BODY COOL DOWN** (see pages 138–9).

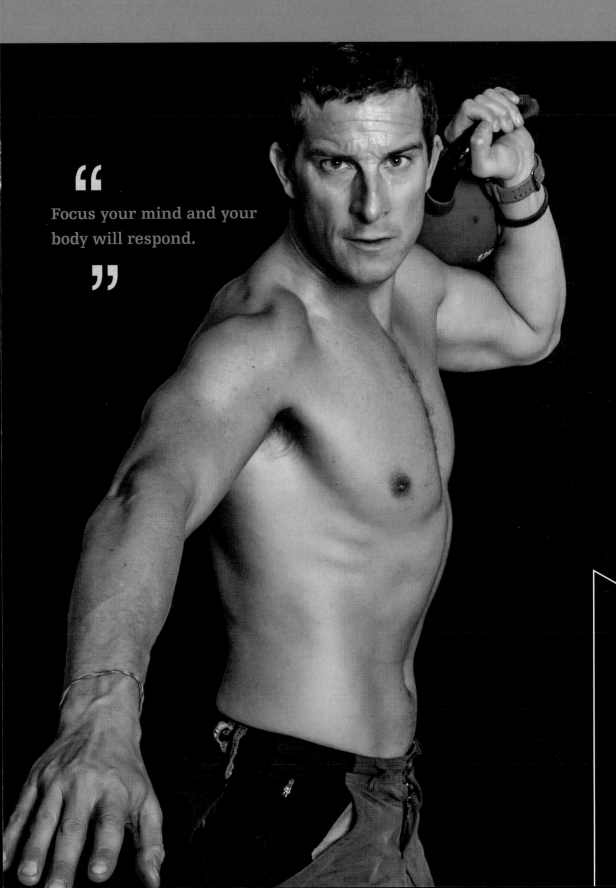

"
Focus your mind and your body will respond.
"

BODYWEIGHT WORKOUT ONE
WHOLE BODY; EMPHASIS ON UPPER BODY

TIME: 15 MINUTES OR 30 MINUTES

COMPLETE THE FOLLOWING BLOCKS OF EXERCISES ONCE FOR A 15-MINUTE WORKOUT OR TWICE FOR A 30-MINUTE WORKOUT.

EQUIPMENT: PULL-UP BAR/BRANCH, MAT

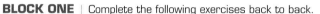

COMPLETE YOUR **BODYWEIGHT WARM-UP** (see pages 132–3).

BLOCK ONE | Complete the following exercises back to back.

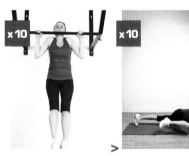 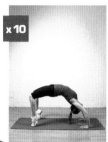 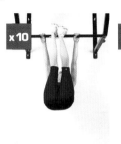 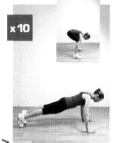

x10 — Pull-ups (see page 90) > x10 — Dragon Push-ups (see page 95) > x10 — Toes to Bar (see page 93) > x10 — Reverse Push-ups (see page 89) > x10 — Bear Leap and Reaches (see page 67)

REST FOR 1 MINUTE

BLOCK TWO | Complete the following exercises back to back.

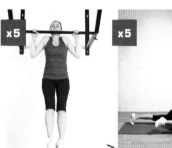 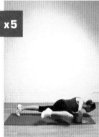 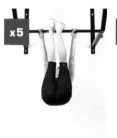 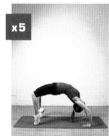 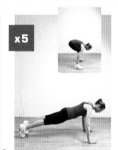

x5 — Pull-ups (see page 90) > x5 — Dragon Push-ups (see page 95) > x5 — Toes to Bar (see page 93) > x5 — Reverse Push-ups (see page 89) > x5 — Bear Leap and Reaches (see page 67)

REST FOR 2 MINUTES

BLOCK THREE | Complete the following exercises back to back.

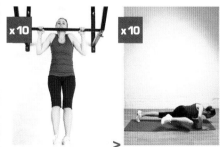 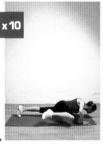 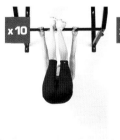 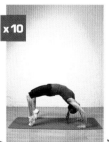 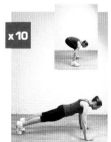

x10 — Pull-ups (see page 90) > x10 — Dragon Push-ups (see page 95) > x10 — Toes to Bar (see page 93) > x10 — Reverse Push-ups (see page 89) > x10 — Bear Leap and Reaches (see page 67)

REST FOR 1 MINUTE

BLOCK FOUR | Complete the following exercises back to back.

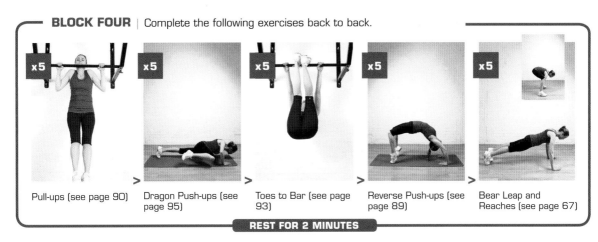

x5	**x5**	**x5**	**x5**	**x5**
Pull-ups (see page 90)	Dragon Push-ups (see page 95)	Toes to Bar (see page 93)	Reverse Push-ups (see page 89)	Bear Leap and Reaches (see page 67)

REST FOR 2 MINUTES

BLOCK FIVE | Complete each of the following exercises for 30 seconds.
Move from one exercise to the other without a rest.

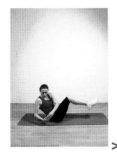 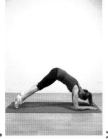 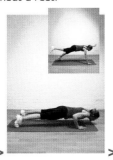 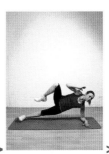 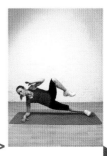

Russian Twists (see page 73)	Bear V Planks (see page 63)	Tri to Superman Push (see page 98)	Spider Side Plank, right (see page 64)	Spider Side Plank, left

REST FOR 2 MINUTES

RECOVER AND COMPLETE A **FULL-BODY COOL DOWN** (see pages 138–9).

BODYWEIGHT WORKOUT TWO
WHOLE BODY; EMPHASIS ON LOWER BODY

TIME: 10 MINUTES, 20 MINUTES OR 30 MINUTES

COMPLETE THE SEQUENCES ONCE FOR A 10-MINUTE WORKOUT; TWICE FOR A 20-MINUTE WORKOUT; THREE TIMES FOR A 30-MINUTE WORKOUT.

EQUIPMENT: MAT

COMPLETE YOUR **BODYWEIGHT WARM-UP** [see pages 132–3].

BLOCK ONE | Complete the following exercises back to back.

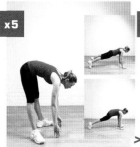
Inchworm to alternating Bear Leaps (see pages 70 and 67)

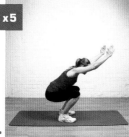
Squats with Arms (see page 80)

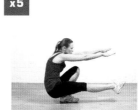
Pistol Squats, right (see page 78)

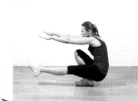
Pistol Squats, left

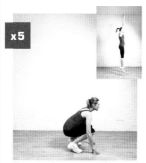
Burpees (see page 86)

■ | Rest for 30 seconds and repeat.

REST FOR 1 MINUTE

BLOCK TWO | Complete each of the following exercises for 20 seconds and rest for 10 seconds between exercises.

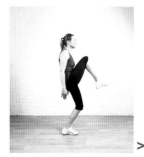
High Knees (see page 76)

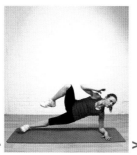
Spider Side Plank, right (see page 64)

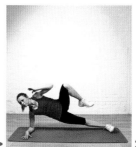
Spider Side Plank, left

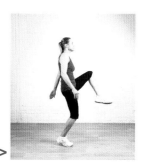
High Knees with Arms (see variation, page 76)

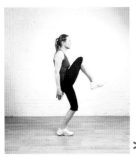

High Knees

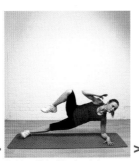

Spider Side Plank, right

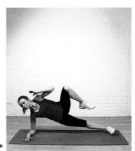

Spider Side Plank, left

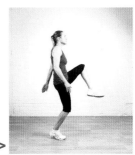

High Knees with Arms

REST FOR 1 MINUTE

BLOCK THREE | Complete the following exercises back to back for 30 seconds.

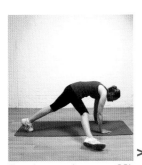

Grasshoppers (see page 68)

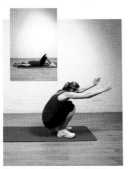

Squat to Abdominal Roll-out to Standing (see page 81)

REST FOR 1 MINUTE

BLOCK FOUR | Complete each of the following exercises for 45 seconds.
Move from one exercise to the other without a rest.

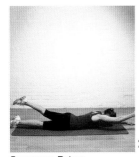

Superman Raises
(see page 96)

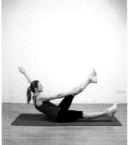

Cross Crunches
(see page 72)

> " Don't just go through the
> motions – give 100 per cent! "

REST FOR 1 MINUTE

WHEN YOU HAVE FINISHED YOUR ENTIRE WORKOUT, RECOVER
AND COMPLETE A **FULL-BODY COOL DOWN** (see pages 138–9).

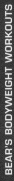

BODYWEIGHT WORKOUT THREE
WHOLE BODY; EMPHASIS ON CORE

COMPLETE THE FOLLOWING BLOCKS OF EXERCISES ONCE FOR A 10-MINUTE WORKOUT; TWICE FOR 20-MINUTE WORKOUT; THREE TIMES FOR A 30-MINUTE WORKOUT.

TIME: 10 MINUTES, 20 MINUTES OR 30 MINUTES

EQUIPMENT: PULL-UP BAR/BRANCH, MAT

COMPLETE YOUR **BODYWEIGHT WARM-UP** (see pages 132–3).

BLOCK ONE | Complete the following sequence of exercises.
Work for 20 seconds and rest for 10 seconds between exercises.

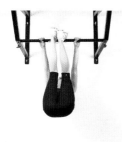
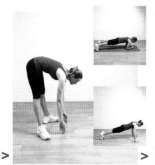
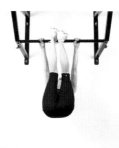
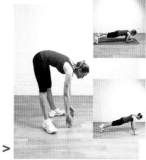

Toes to Bar (see page 93)   Inchworm to Low–High Plank (see pages 70 and 62)   Toes to Bar   Inchworm to Low–High Plank

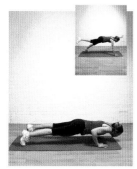
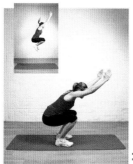
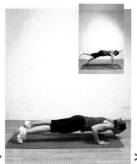
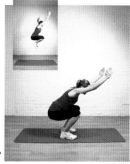

Tri to Superman Push (see page 98)   Bear Squats (see page 82)   Tri to Superman Push   Bear Squats

REST FOR 30 SECONDS

BLOCK TWO | Complete the following sequence of exercises.
Work for 20 seconds and rest for 10 seconds between exercises.

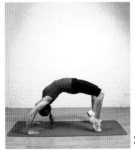 > 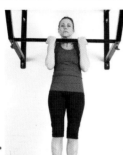 > 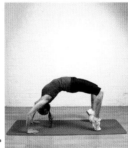 >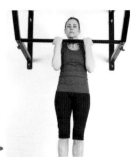

Reverse Push-up (see page 89) > Narrow Pull-ups, underhand grip (see page 90) > Reverse Push Up > Narrow Pull-ups, underhand grip

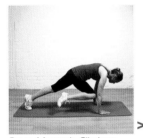 > 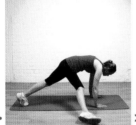 > 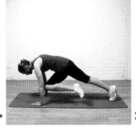 >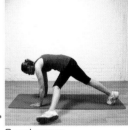

Cross Mountain Climbers (see page 66) > Grasshoppers (see page 68) > Cross Mountain Climbers > Grasshoppers

REST FOR 30 SECONDS

BLOCK THREE | Complete the following exercise for 1 minute.

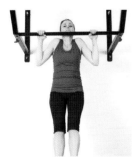

Pull-ups (see page 90)

"
Pull-ups are seen as one of the ultimate fitness tests. They're tough! But remember: you don't have to be good at them at the start, but you do have to start in order to get better!
"

REST FOR 1 MINUTE

WHEN YOU HAVE FINISHED YOUR ENTIRE WORKOUT, RECOVER AND COMPLETE A **FULL-BODY COOL DOWN** (see pages 138–9).

COMPLETE THE SEQUENCES ONCE FOR A 10-MINUTE WORKOUT; TWICE FOR A 20-MINUTE WORKOUT; THREE TIMES FOR A 30-MINUTE WORKOUT.

TIME: 10 MINUTES, 20 MINUTES OR 30 MINUTES

EQUIPMENT: MAT

COMPLETE YOUR **PRIMAL POWER STRETCH WARM-UP** (see pages 134–5).

BLOCK ONE | Complete the following standing-strength sequence. Hold each pose for 45 seconds. Repeat the sequence 4 times (2 times on your left-hand side; 2 times on your right-hand side) to complete the exercise block.

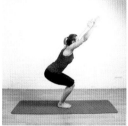
Standing Chair (see page 112)

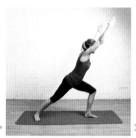
Warrior One (see page 114)

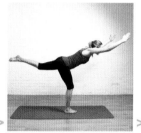
Warrior Lunge and Reach (see page 118)

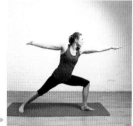
Warrior Two (see page 116)

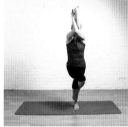
Eagle Pose (see page 121)

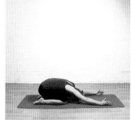
Extended Bear Pose

Connect with your breath. Use your exhale to settle deeper into the pose in both body and mind.

REST: PAUSE FOR 5 BREATHS IN EXTENDED BEAR POSE (SEE PAGE 125).

BLOCK TWO | Complete the following core-strength sequence. Hold each pose for 30 seconds. Repeat the sequence 3 times to complete the exercise block.

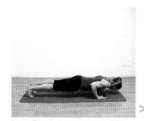
Low Plank (see page 105)

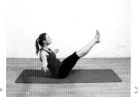
Boat Pose (see page 110)

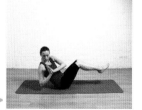
Russian Prayer Twist (see page 111)

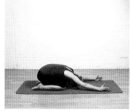
Extended Bear Pose

REST: PAUSE FOR 5 BREATHS IN EXTENDED BEAR POSE (SEE PAGE 125).

■ | Extend through to Forward Fold (see page 104) and rise into Mountain Pose, prayer hands (see page 102) to complete the workout.

WHEN YOU HAVE FINISHED YOUR ENTIRE WORKOUT, RECOVER AND COMPLETE A **FULL-BODY COOL DOWN** (see pages 138–9).

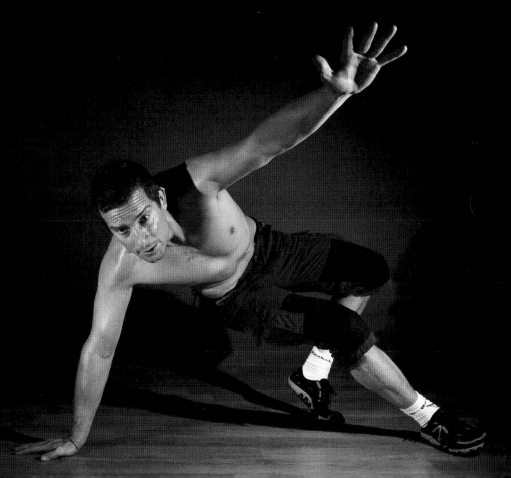

> It feels amazing to be able to move like this – with balance and control. This type of exercise is critical in my line of work – speed, agility and strength combined.

WHOLE BODY; EMPHASIS ON SPINAL MOBILITY

COMPLETE THE SEQUENCES ONCE FOR A 10-MINUTE WORKOUT; TWICE FOR A 20-MINUTE WORKOUT; THREE TIMES FOR A 30-MINUTE WORKOUT.

TIME: 10 MINUTES, 20 MINUTES OR 30 MINUTES

EQUIPMENT: MAT

COMPLETE YOUR **PRIMAL POWER STRETCH WARM-UP** (see pages 134–5).

BLOCK ONE | Complete the following block of exercises once for a 10-minute workout; twice for 20-minute workout; three times for a 30-minute workout.

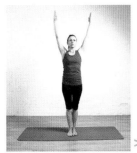
Extended Mountain Pose (see page 103)

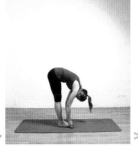
Forward Fold, deep (see page 104)

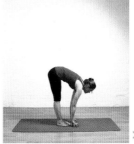
Forward Fold, eye gaze forward

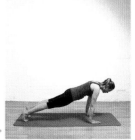
High Plank (see page 105)

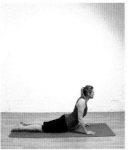
Up Dog (see page 106)

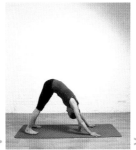
Down Dog (see page 107)

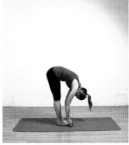
Forward Fold, deep

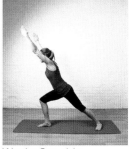
Warrior One, right (see page 114)

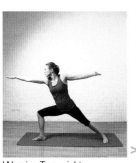
Warrior Two, right (see page 116)

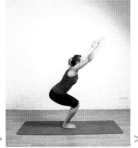
Standing Chair (see page 112)

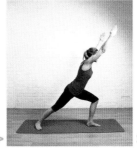
Warrior One, left

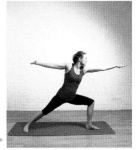
Warrior Two, left

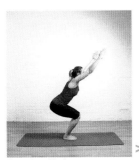

Standing Chair

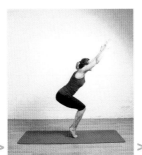

Advanced Standing Chair, on toes

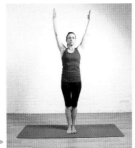

Extended Mountain Pose

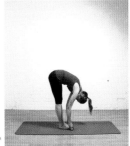

Forward Fold, deep

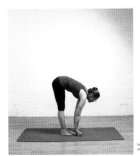

Forward Fold, eye gaze forward

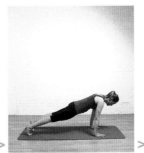

High Plank

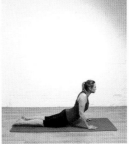

Up Dog

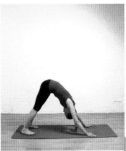

Down Dog

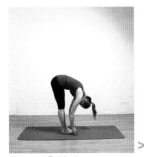

Forward Fold, deep

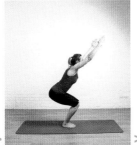

Standing Chair

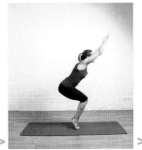

Advanced Standing Chair, on toes

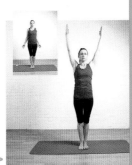

Extended Mountain Pose to Mountain Pose

WHEN YOU HAVE FINISHED YOUR ENTIRE WORKOUT, RECOVER AND COMPLETE A **FULL-BODY COOL DOWN** (see pages 138–9).

TIME: 30 MINUTES

COMPLETE THE FOLLOWING BLOCKS OF EXERCISES
FOR A 30-MINUTE WORKOUT.

EQUIPMENT: MAT

COMPLETE YOUR **PRIMAL POWER STRETCH WARM-UP** (see pages 134–5).

BLOCK ONE | Complete the following sequence of exercises.
Hold each pose for 20 seconds then use the 10 seconds' rest to transition
into the next pose or hold the transition pose where cued.

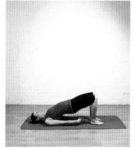

Hip Bridge (see page 113)

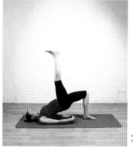

Single-leg Hip Bridge, left
and right (see page 113)

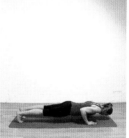

Low Plank (see page 105)

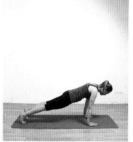

High Plank (see page 105)

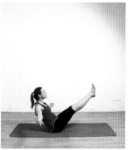

Boat Pose (see page 110)

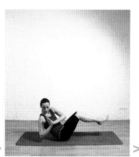

Russian Prayer Twist in
transition (see page 111)

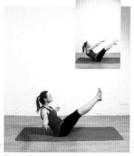

Boat Pose to V Sit-up (see
page 71)

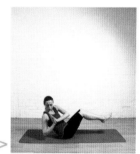

Russian Prayer Twist in
transition

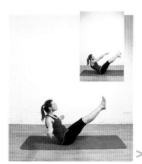

Boat Pose to V Sit-up

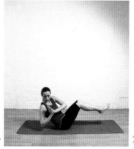

Russian Prayer Twist in
transition

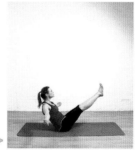

Boat Pose

BLOCK TWO | Complete the following sequence of exercises. Hold each pose for 20 seconds, then use the 10 seconds' rest to transition into the next pose or hold the transition pose where cued.

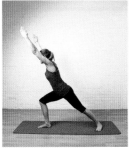

Warrior One, right (see page 114)

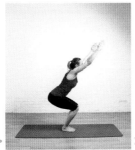

Standing Chair, extended arms (see page 112)

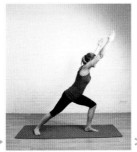

Warrior One left

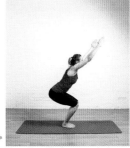

Standing Chair, extended arms

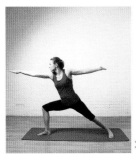

Warrior Two, right (see page 116)

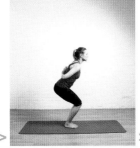

Standing Chair, prayer arms behind back

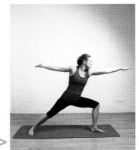

Warrior Two, left

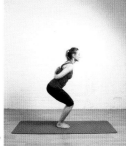

Standing Chair, prayer arms behind back

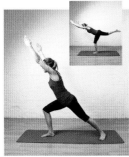

Warrior One, right, into Warrior Lunge and Reach, right (see page 118)

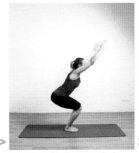

Standing Chair, extended arms

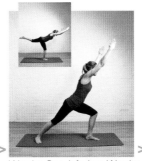

Warrior One, left, into Warrior Lunge and Reach, left

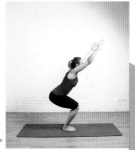

Standing Chair, extended arms

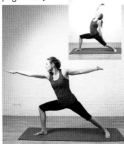

Warrior Two, right, to Reverse Warrior Two, right (see page 117)

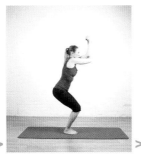

Standing Chair, eagle arms (see page 112)

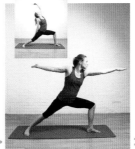

Warrior Two, left, to Reverse Warrior Two, left

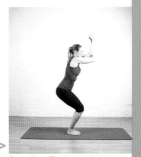

Standing Chair, eagle arms

CONTINUES OVERLEAF

CONTINUED FROM PAGE 163

BLOCK THREE | Complete the following sequence of exercises. Hold each pose for 20 seconds, then use the 10 seconds' rest to transition into the next pose or hold the transition pose where cued.

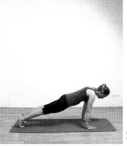 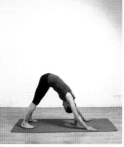 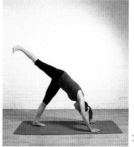 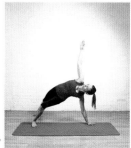

High Plank (see page 105) Start to lift hips towards ceiling and transition to:

Down Dog (see page 107) Lift right leg off floor and transition to:

Split Down Dog (see page 108) Bend right knee and bring heel towards buttocks.

Hold Bent Knee Split Down Dog or transition to Wild Thing (see page 126)

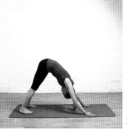 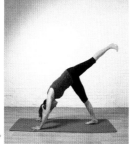 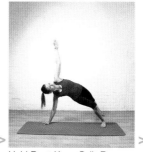 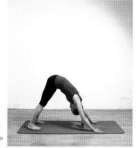

Transition back to: Down Dog Lift left leg off floor and transition to:

Split Down Dog Bend left knee and bring heel towards buttocks.

Hold Bent Knee Split Dog or transition to Wild Thing. Transition back to:

Down Dog

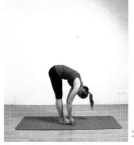 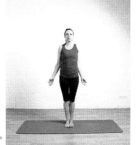

Transition back to Forward Fold (see page 104)

and then to Mountain Pose (see page 102)

> **"**
> Make each pose powerful by committing to mastering your technique and aiming to improve it further with each workout.
> **"**

REST FOR 5 BREATHS IN MOUNTAIN POSE (SEE PAGE 102).

BLOCK FOUR | Complete the following standing-strength sequence to make one round. Hold each pose for 45 seconds with no rest between exercises. Repeat the sequence 5 times to complete the exercise block.

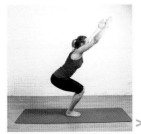

Standing Chair (see page 112)

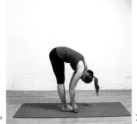

Forward Fold (see page 104) Step out to:

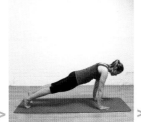

High Plank (see page 105) Step in to:

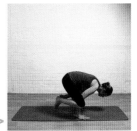

Crow Pose (see page 122) Step back to:

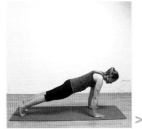

High Plank
Step in to:

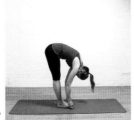

Forward Fold

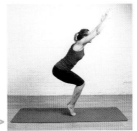

Advanced Standing Chair Pose, on toes (see page 112)

REST: EXTEND INTO MOUNTAIN POSE FOR 5 BREATHS.

BLOCK FIVE | Complete the following core-strength sequence. Hold each pose for 60 seconds with no rest between exercises.

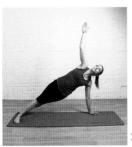

Side Stand to T-Stand, right and left (see page 124)

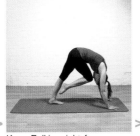

Knee Pull-in, right (see page 109)

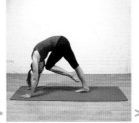

Knee Pull-in, left

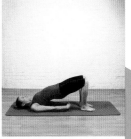

Hip Bridge (see page 113)

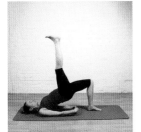

Single-leg Hip Bridge, right and left (see page 113)

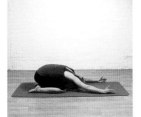

Extended Bear Pose (see page 125)

REST: PAUSE FOR 5 BREATHS IN EXTENDED BEAR POSE (SEE PAGE 125).

■ | Extend through to Forward Fold (see page 104) and rise into Mountain Pose, prayer hands (see page 102) to complete the workout.

WHEN YOU HAVE FINISHED YOUR ENTIRE WORKOUT, RECOVER AND COMPLETE A **FULL-BODY COOL DOWN** (see pages 138–9).

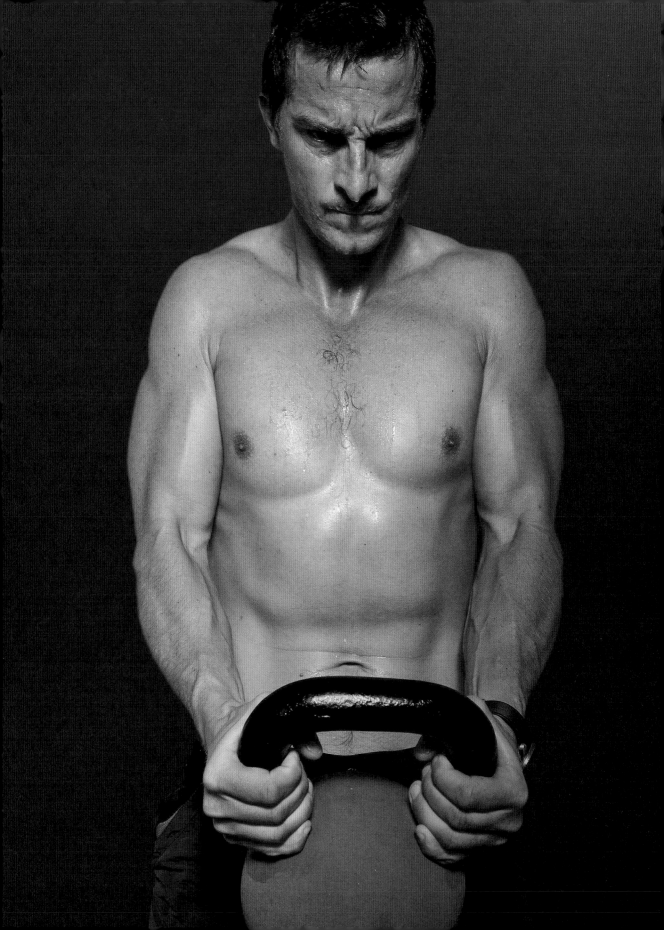

BEAR'S HERO WORKOUTS

Welcome to my ultimate challenge: the Hero workouts. I love to do these with my crew and friends and they are designed for 10, 20 and 30 minutes of maximum body-shock!

Prepare to dig deep, work hard and get sweaty! Be warned: you may feel a little exhausted at the end, but after 30 minutes or less you will be energized and ready to tackle anything life throws at you!

Remember to focus on technique.
Those who dig the deepest get
the best results.

HERO WORKOUT ONE

DISCIPLINE: KETTLEBELL, BODYWEIGHT, PRIMAL POWER STRETCH

TIME: APPROX. 30 MINUTES

EQUIPMENT: PULL-UP BAR/BRANCH, KETTLEBELLS, MAT

COMPLETE **HERO WARM-UP** (see pages 136–7).

BLOCK ONE | Complete the following sequence of exercises.
Work for 20 seconds and rest for 10 seconds between exercises.

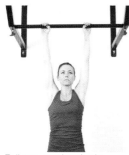 > 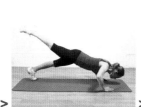 > 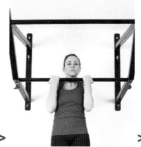 >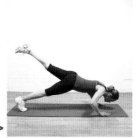

| Pull-ups, overhand grip (see page 90) | Push-ups, right leg elevated (see page 94) | Pull-ups, narrow hand grip | Push-ups, left leg elevated |

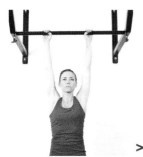 > 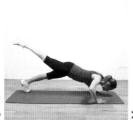 > 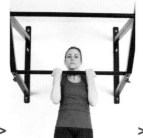 >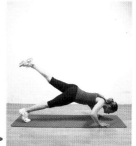

| Pull-ups, overhand grip | Push-ups, right leg elevated | Pull-ups, narrow hand grip | Push-ups, left leg elevated |

REST FOR I MINUTE

BLOCK TWO | Complete the following sequence of exercises.
Work for 20 seconds and rest for 10 seconds between exercises.

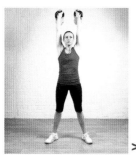 > 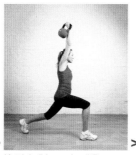 > 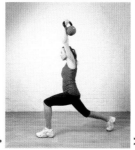 >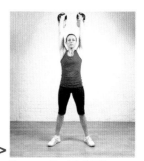

| Two-arm Kettlebell Military Press (see page 46) | Kettlebell Lunge and Press, right (see page 48) | Kettlebell Lunge and Press, left | Two-arm Kettlebell Military Press |

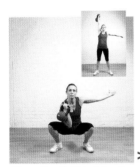

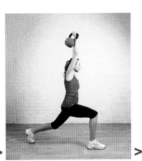

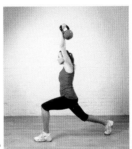

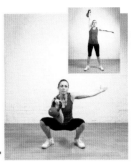

Alternating Kettlebell Front Squat to Press, right and left (see page 44)

Kettlebell Lunge and Press, right (see page 48)

Kettlebell Lunge and Press, left

Alternating Kettlebell Front Squat to Press, right and left

REST FOR I MINUTE

BLOCK THREE | Complete the following sequence of exercises. Work for 20 seconds and rest for 10 seconds between exercises.

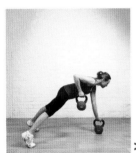

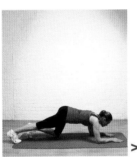

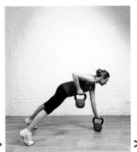

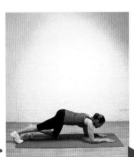

Kettlebell Power Plank with Renegade Row (see page 43)

Crawl Plank (see page 61)

Kettlebell Power Plank with Renegade Row

Crawl Plank

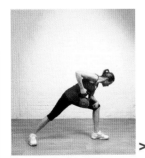

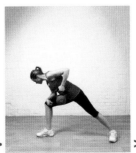

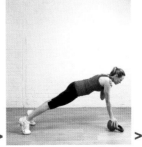

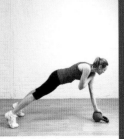

One-arm Kettlebell Row, right (see page 40)

One-arm Kettlebell Row, left

Kettlebell Single-arm Plank, right (see page 41)

Kettlebell Single-arm Plank, left

REST FOR 1 MINUTE

CONTINUES OVERLEAF

BEAR'S HERO WORKOUTS

BLOCK FOUR | Complete the following sequence of exercises.
Work for 20 seconds and rest for 10 seconds between exercises.

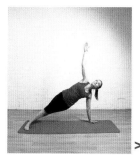 > 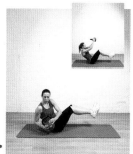 > 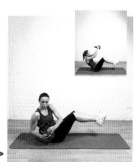 >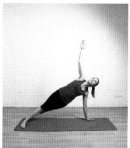

Alternating Side Stand to T Stand, right and left (see page 124)

Bear Twist and Press (see page 55)

Alternating Side Stand to T Stand, right and left

Bear Twist and Press

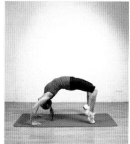 > 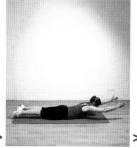 > 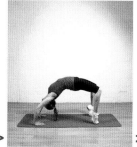 >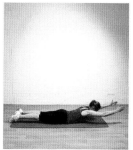

Reverse Push-ups (see page 89)

Dorsal Raises (see page 99)

Reverse Push-ups

Dorsal Raises

REST FOR 1 MINUTE

BLOCK FIVE | Complete the following sequence of exercises.
Complete as many rounds as possible in 3 minutes.

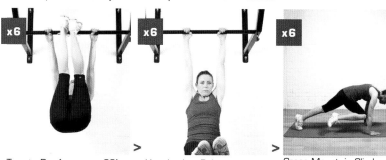

x6   x6   x6

Toes to Bar (see page 93) > Hanging Leg Raises (see page 92) > Cross Mountain Climbers with a Push-up (see page 66)

REST FOR 1 MINUTE

RECOVER AND COMPLETE A **FULL-BODY COOL DOWN** (see pages 138–9).

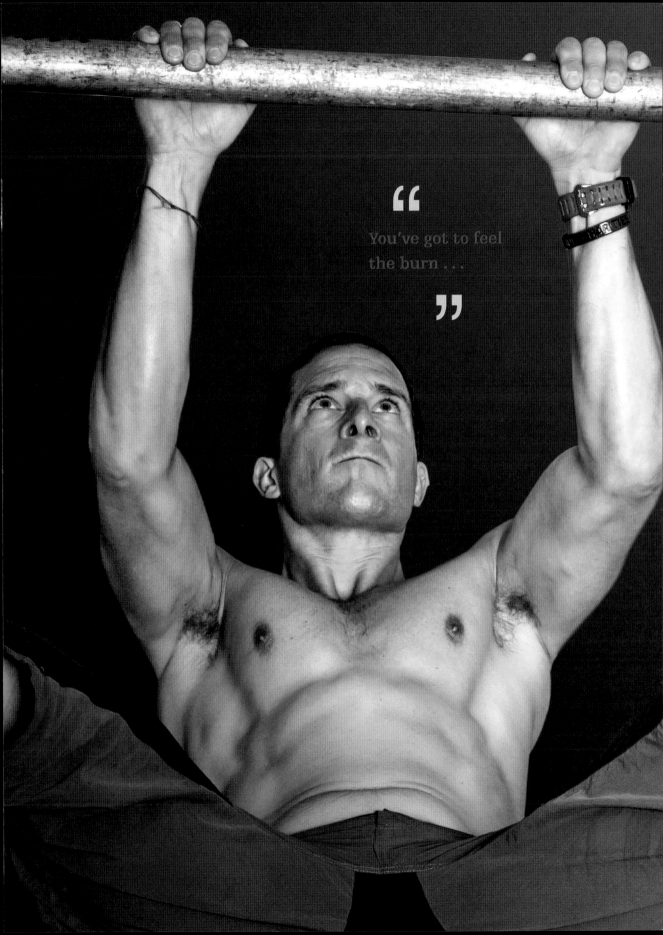

" You've got to feel the burn ... "

HERO WORKOUT TWO

DISCIPLINE: BODYWEIGHT, PRIMAL POWER STRETCH

TIME: APPROX. 30 MINUTES

EQUIPMENT: MAT

COMPLETE YOUR **HERO WARM-UP** (see pages 136–7).

BLOCK ONE | Complete each of the following exercises for 60 seconds. Rest for 15 seconds between exercises.

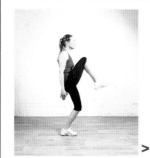 > 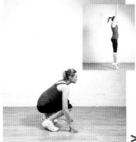 > 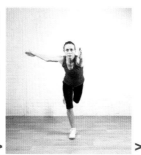 >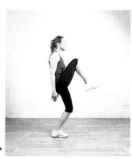

Sprint Run, on the spot | Burpees (see page 86) | Ice Skaters (see page 75) | Sprint Run, on the spot

REST FOR 2 MINUTES

BLOCK TWO | Complete the following core- and leg-strength Primal Power Stretch sequence. Complete each pose for 30 seconds. Repeat the sequence twice.

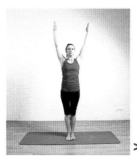 > 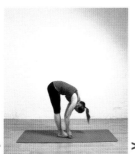 > 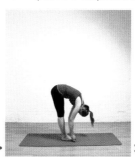 >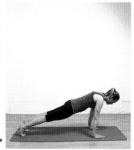

Extended Mountain Pose (see page 103) | Forward Fold, deep (see page 104) | Forward Fold, deep | High Plank (see page 105)

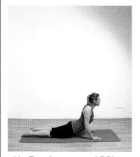 > 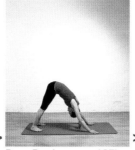 > 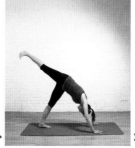 >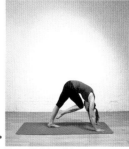

Up Dog (see page 106) | Down Dog (see page 107) | Split Down Dog, right leg lifts (see page 108) | Knee Pull-in, right (see page 109)

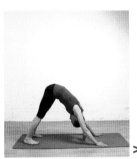 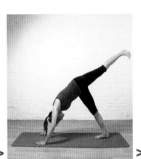 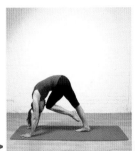 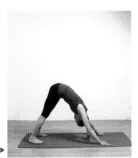

Down Dog > Split Down Dog, left leg lifts > Knee Pull-in, left > Down Dog

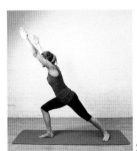 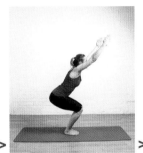 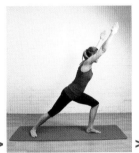 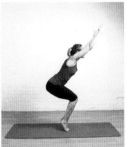

Warrior One, right (see page 114) > Standing Chair (see page 112) > Warrior One, left > Advanced Standing Chair, on toes

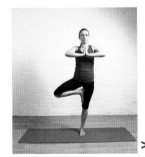 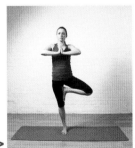 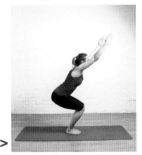

Tree Pose, right (see page 120) > Tree Pose, left > Standing Chair

ONCE YOU HAVE COMPLETED THE SEQUENCE TWICE, REST FOR 1 MINUTE.

RECOVER AND COMPLETE A **FULL-BODY COOL DOWN**
STARTING WITH SEATED HAMSTRING STRETCH (see page 139).

HERO WORKOUT THREE

DISCIPLINE: KETTLEBELL, BODYWEIGHT, PRIMAL POWER STRETCH

COMPLETE THE FOLLOWING EXERCISE BLOCKS FOR A 20-MINUTE EXPRESS WHOLE-BODY WORKOUT.

TIME: A MORE INTENSE 20 MINUTES

EQUIPMENT: KETTLEBELLS, MAT

COMPLETE **HERO WARM-UP** (see pages 136–7).

BLOCK ONE | Complete the following sequence of exercises to make one round. Repeat as many rounds as possible in 8 minutes.
You must hit fatigue towards the last round. If you feel you can do more, increase your kettlebell weight.

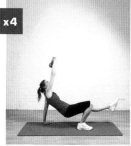

Kettlebell Turkish Get-up Half, right (see page 57)

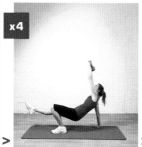

Kettlebell Turkish Get-up Half, left

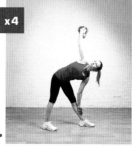

Kettlebell Windmill, right (see page 51)

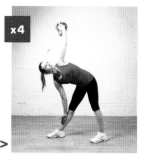

Kettlebell Windmill, left

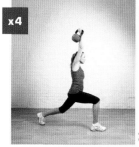

Kettlebell Lunge and Press, right (see page 48)

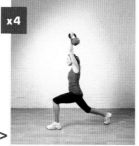

Kettlebell Lunge and Press, left

BLOCK TWO | Complete the following sequence of poses back to back.
Hold each one for 45 seconds with no rest in between poses.

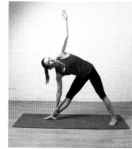

Triangle, right (see page 119)

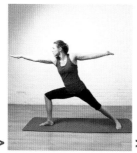

Warrior Two, right (see page 116)

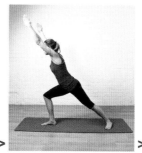

Warrior One, right (see page 114)

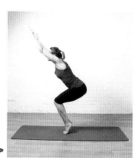

Advanced Standing Chair, on toes (see page 112)

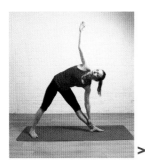

Triangle, left

>

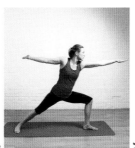

Warrior Two, left

>

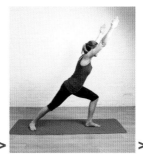

Warrior One, left

>

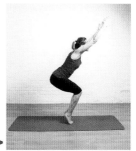

Advanced Standing Chair, on toes

REST FOR I MINUTE

BLOCK THREE | Complete each of the following exercises for 1 minute back to back with no rest in between exercises.

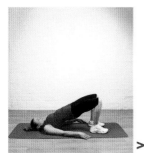

Hip Bridge Dips (see page 85)

>

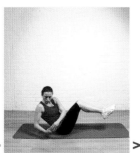

Russian Prayer Twists (see page 111)

>

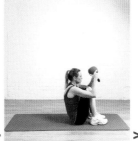

Abdominal Pull-ins (see page 38)

>

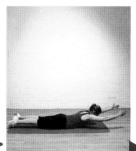

Dorsal Raises (see page 99)

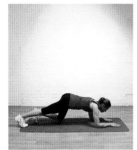

Crawl Plank (see page 61)

> Less time means you've got to work even harder. Maximum burn, maximum cardio, maximum strength and muscle-shake!

REST FOR 1 MINUTE

RECOVER AND COMPLETE A **FULL-BODY COOL DOWN** (see pages 138–9).

BEAR'S HERO WORKOUTS

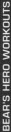

HERO WORKOUT FOUR

DISCIPLINE: KETTLEBELL, BODYWEIGHT, PRIMAL POWER STRETCH

COMPLETE THE FOLLOWING BLOCKS OF EXERCISES ONCE FOR A 10-MINUTE WORKOUT; TWICE FOR A 20-MINUTE WORKOUT; THREE TIMES FOR A 30-MINUTE WORKOUT. THE SHORTER THE TIME, THE HARDER YOU HAVE TO WORK!

TIME: 10 MINUTES, 20 MINUTES OR 30 MINUTES

EQUIPMENT: KETTLEBELLS, MAT

COMPLETE **HERO WARM-UP** (see page 136–7).

BLOCK ONE | Complete each of the following exercises for 20 seconds. Rest for 10 seconds in between exercises.

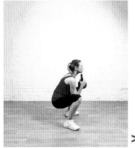

Goblet Squat (see page 45)

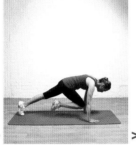

Mountain Climbers (see page 65)

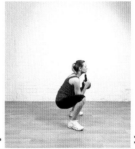

Goblet Squat

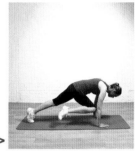

Cross Mountain Climbers (see page 66)

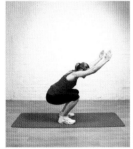

Squat with Arms (see page 80)

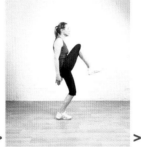

High Knees (see page 76)

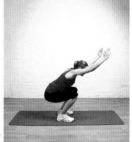

Squat with Arms

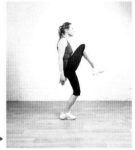

High Knees

REST FOR 30 SECONDS

BLOCK TWO | Complete the following sequence of exercises to make one round. Repeat as many rounds as possible in 3 minutes.

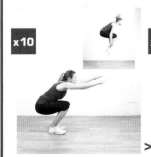

x10

Bear Tucks (see page 84)

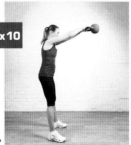

x10

Double-hand Swings (see page 31)

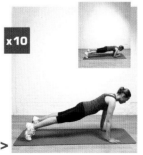

x10

High to Low Planks (see page 62)

BEAR'S HERO WORKOUTS

BLOCK THREE | Complete each of the following exercises for 30 seconds with no rest in between exercises.

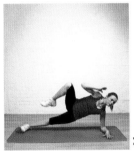

Spider Side Plank, right (see page 64)

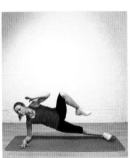

Spider Side Plank, left

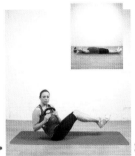

Kettlebell 3-point Russian Twist (see page 56)

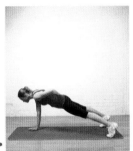

Single-hand Plank, right (see page 62)

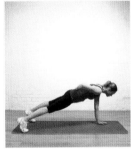

Single-hand Plank, left

> **"**
> Your ability is limitless – do more, train better, fuel well, recover and be fit.
> **"**

REST FOR 30 SECONDS

RECOVER AND COMPLETE A **FULL-BODY COOL DOWN** (see pages 138–9).

HERO WORKOUT FIVE

DISCIPLINE: KETTLEBELL, BODYWEIGHT

COMPLETE THE FOLLOWING EXERCISES ONCE FOR A 10-MINUTE WORKOUT; TWICE FOR A 20-MINUTE WORKOUT; THREE TIMES FOR A 30-MINUTE WORKOUT. THE SHORTER THE TIME, THE HARDER YOU HAVE TO WORK!

TIME: 10 MINUTES, 20 MINUTES OR 30 MINUTES

EQUIPMENT: KETTLEBELLS, MAT, PULL-UP BAR/BRANCH

COMPLETE **HERO WARM-UP** (see pages 136–7).

BLOCK ONE | Complete each of the following exercises for 20 seconds. Rest for 10 seconds in between exercises.

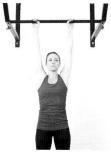

Pull-ups (see page 90)

>

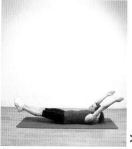

Bear Tucks (see page 84)

>

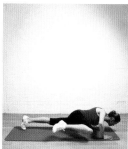

Abdominal Rocks (see page 74)

>

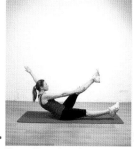

Dragon Push-up (see page 95)

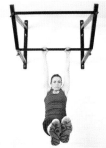

Hanging Leg Raises (see page 92), drop to

>

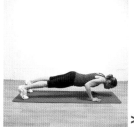

Narrow Push-ups (see page 98)

>

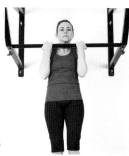

Cross Crunches (see page 72)

>

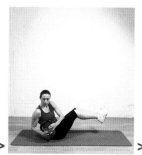

Narrow Pull-ups (see page 90)

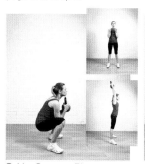

Goblet Squat to Bicep to Double-hand Military Press (see pages 45 and 49)

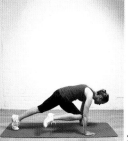

Cross Mountain Climbers (see page 66)

>

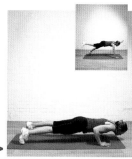

Kettlebell Russian Twists (see pages 54–5)

>

Tri to Superman Push (see page 98)

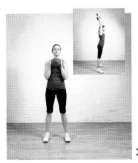 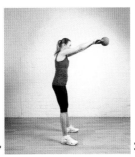 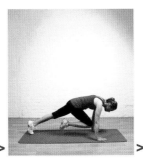 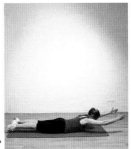

Bicep to Double-hand Military Press

> Double-hand Swings (see page 31)

> Mountain Climbers (see page 65)

> Dorsal Raises (see page 99)

REST FOR 1 MINUTE

RECOVER AND COMPLETE A **FULL-BODY COOL DOWN** (see pages 138–9).

"

Out of breath, sweaty, feeling the burn? Yes? Great, it's working!

"

6 | DESIGNING A WORKOUT UNIQUE TO YOU

'Form, endeavour, consistency – the building blocks of great athletes.'

NOW YOU'RE FAMILIAR WITH THE EXERCISES AND THE STYLE OF TRAINING, YOU'RE READY TO PROGRESS AND BUILD YOUR OWN SESSIONS.

IN THIS SECTION WE'LL SHOW YOU HOW TO PUT TOGETHER YOUR OWN PERSONALIZED, FOCUSED WORKOUT TO MEET YOUR INDIVIDUAL GOALS BY BUILDING A SEQUENCE OF EXERCISE BLOCKS.

The examples of blocks that follow are listed by training discipline and the time it takes to complete them. This is your chance to design a personalized and unique workout specific to your exercise goals, and here is how you do it:

1. Decide on the workout training discipline: Kettlebell or Bodyweight.
2. Pick a warm-up specific to your training discipline (see pages 130–5).
3. Select your exercise blocks based on the following:

- Target areas – *for example, whole body.*
- Training method (see page 12) – *tabata, AMRAP or density.*
- Time – *for example, 2 x 4-minute blocks if you have 15 minutes available (remember to factor in your warm-up and cool-down time).*

4. Include a cool down to complete your personalized workout (see pages 138–9).

Opposite is what your unique workout may look like.

TRAINING DISCIPLINE	KETTLEBELL TRAINING
Warm-up: **approx. 3–6 minutes**	**Kettlebell Warm-up (see pages 130–1)** ■ 8 Shoulder Rolls, forwards and backwards ■ 8 Arm Circles, forwards and backwards ■ 8 Hip Circles, right ■ 8 Hip Circles, left ■ 8 Hip Drives ■ 8 Squats with Hug and Diagonal Open ■ 8 Knees to Chests ■ 4 Lunges with side bend, right ■ 4 Lunges with side bend, left ■ 4 Lunges with rotation, right ■ 4 Lunges with rotation, left ■ 8 Hip Bridge Dips ■ 8 Kettlebell Deadlifts ■ 8 Standing Abdominal 8s ■ 8 alternating Abdominal 8s to Woodchops
Target Areas	Whole body and core
Training Methods	Tabata and AMRAP
Time	15 minutes (including warm-up and cool-down)
Exercise Block One Discipline: Kettlebell Tabata Three: pure core sequence Time: 4 minutes	Complete each of the following exercises for 20 seconds. Rest for 10 seconds in between exercises. ■ Kettlebell Power Plank with Row, right (see page 42) ■ Kettlebell Power Plank with Row, left ■ Kettlebell Russian Twists (see pages 54–5) ■ Kettlebell Power Plank with Row, right ■ Kettlebell Power Plank with Row, left ■ Kettlebell Russian Twists ■ Kettlebell Single-arm Plank (right) (see page 41) ■ Kettlebell Single-arm Plank (left)
Exercise Block Two Discipline: Kettlebell AMRAP One: whole body Time: 5 minutes	Complete the following sequence of exercises. Complete as many rounds as possible in 5 minutes. ■ 4 Bicep to Double-hand Military Presses (see page 49) ■ 4 Abdominal Crunch to Standings (see page 39) ■ 4 Goblet Squats (see page 45) ■ 4 Kettlebell Power Planks with Renegade Row (see page 43)
Cool down: **approx. 3–6 minutes**	Full-body stretch

Here is the point where you can have some fun building your personalized workouts. Below are a number of exercise blocks from the Kettlebell and Bodyweight disciplines for you to choose from. They are organized by discipline and by method, so get stuck in and go wild!

KETTLEBELL EXERCISE BLOCKS

KETTLEBELL TABATA

TABATA ONE | Complete each of the following exercises for 20 seconds. Rest for 10 seconds between exercises.

BACK | **TIME: 4 MINUTES**

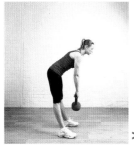

Kettlebell Deadlift (see page 34)

>

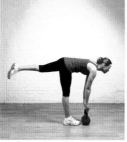

Single-leg Deadlift, right (see page 35)

>

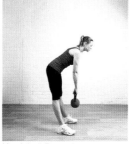

Kettlebell Deadlift

>

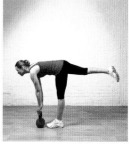

Single-leg Deadlift, left

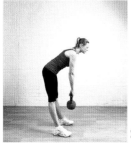

Kettlebell Deadlift

>

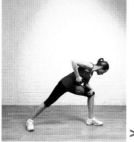

One-arm Kettlebell Row (Warrior Legs), right (see page 40)

>

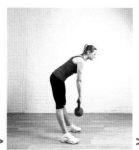

Kettlebell Deadlift

>

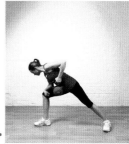

One-arm Kettlebell Row (Warrior Legs), left

TABATA TWO | Complete each of the following exercises for
20 seconds. Rest for 10 seconds between exercises. **WHOLE BODY** | TIME: **4 MINUTES**

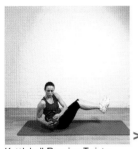
Kettlebell Russian Twists
(see pages 54–5)

>

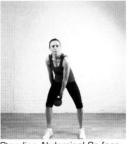
Standing Abdominal 8s (see
page 32)

>

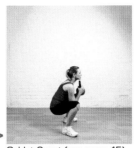
Goblet Squat (see page 45)

>

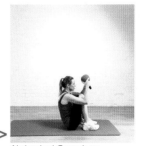
Abdominal Crunch to
Standing (see page 39)

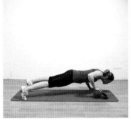
Kettlebell Power Push-ups
(see page 53)

>

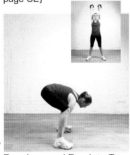
Bear Leap and Reach to Two-
arm Kettlebell Military Press
(see pages 67 and 46)

>

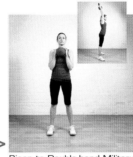
Bicep to Double-hand Military
Press (see page 49)

>

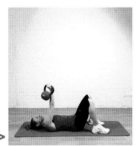
Kettlebell Chest Press (see
page 50)

TABATA THREE | Complete each of the following
exercises for 20 seconds. Rest for 10 seconds between exercises. **PURE CORE SEQUENCE** | TIME: **4 MINUTES**

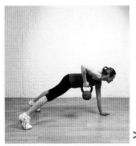
Kettlebell Power Plank with
Row, right (see page 42)

>

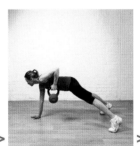
Kettlebell Power Plank with
Row, left

>

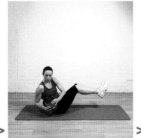
Kettlebell Russian Twists (see
pages 54–5)

>

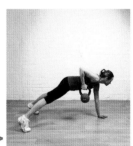
Kettlebell Power Plank with
Row, right

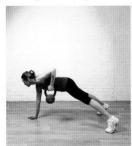
Kettlebell Power Plank with
Row, left

>

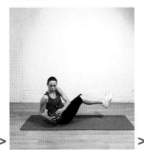
Kettlebell Russian Twists

>

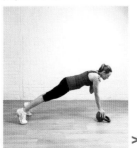
Kettlebell Single-arm Plank,
right (see page 41)

>

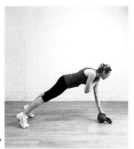
Kettlebell Single-arm Plank,
left

DESIGNING A WORKOUT UNIQUE TO YOU

183

AMRAP ONE | Complete the following sequence of exercises. **WHOLE BODY** | TIME: **8 MINUTES**
Complete as many rounds as possible in 8 minutes.

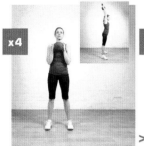
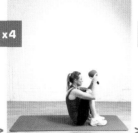
x4

Bicep to Double-hand
Military Presses (see page 49)

>

x4

Abdominal Crunch to
Standings (see page 39)

>

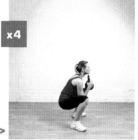
x4

Goblet Squats
(see page 45)

>

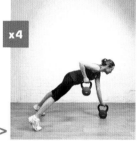
x4

Kettlebell Power Planks with
Renegade Row (see page 43)

AMRAP TWO | Complete the following sequence of exercises. **LOWER BODY** | TIME: **6 MINUTES**
Complete as many rounds as possible in 6 minutes.

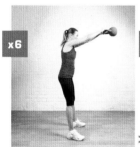
x6

Double-hand Swings
(see page 31)

>

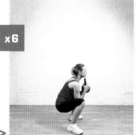
x6

Goblet Squats
(see page 45)

>

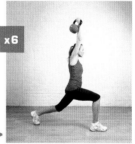
x6

Kettlebell Lunge and Presses,
right (see page 48)

>

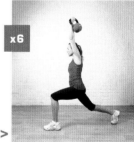
x6

Kettlebell Lunge and
Presses, left

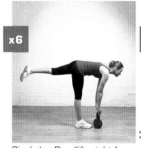
x6

Single-leg Deadlift, right (see
page 35)

>

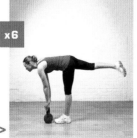
x6

Single-leg Deadlift, left

Train harder than your
last workout and be fitter
than you were.

AMRAP THREE | Complete the following sequence of exercises. Complete as many rounds as possible in 5 minutes.

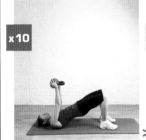

Hip Bridge and Kettlebell Chest Pushes (see page 36)

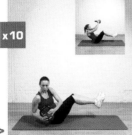

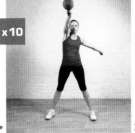

Bear Twists and Presses (see page 55)

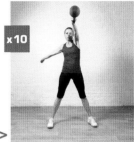

Single-hand Swing, right (see page 30)

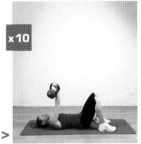

Single-hand Swing, left

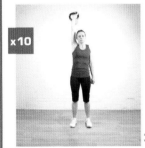

Single-arm Military Press, right (see page 46)

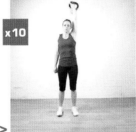

Single-arm Military Press, left

Kettlebell Chest Press (see page 50)

KETTLEBELL DENSITY

DENSITY ONE | Complete the following exercises back to back with no rest.

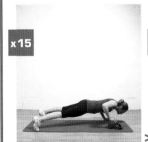

Kettlebell Power Push-ups (see page 53)

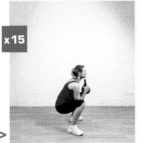

Goblet Squats (see page 45)

DESIGNING A WORKOUT UNIQUE TO YOU

TABATA ONE | Complete each of the following exercises for 20 seconds. Rest for 10 seconds between exercises.

WHOLE BODY | TIME: **4 MINUTES**

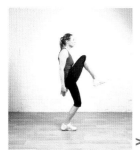

High Knees (see page 76)

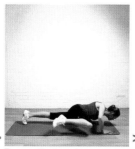

Dragon Push-up (see page 95)

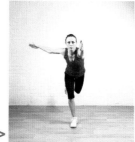

Ice Skaters (see page 75)

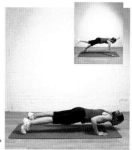

Tri to Superman Push (see page 98)

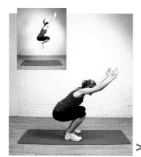

Bear Squats (see page 82)

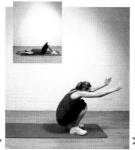

Squat to Abdominal Roll-out to Standing (see page 81)

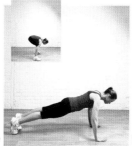

Bear Leap and Reach (see page 67)

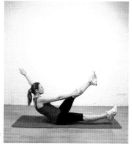

Cross Crunches (see page 72)

TABATA TWO | Complete each of the following exercises for 20 seconds. Rest for 10 seconds between exercises.

CARDIO, LEGS AND CORE | **TIME: 4 MINUTES**

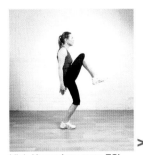

High Knees (see page 76)

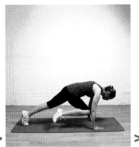

Cross Mountain Climbers (see page 66)

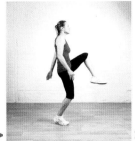

High Knees with Arms (see page 76)

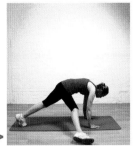

Grasshoppers (see pages 68–9)

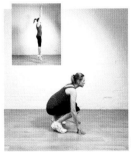

Burpees (see page 86)

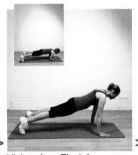

High to Low Plank (see page 62)

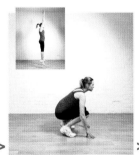

Burpees

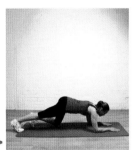

Crawl Plank (see page 61)

TABATA THREE |

UPPER BODY, CORE AND BALANCE | **TIME: 4 MINUTES**

Complete each of the following exercises for 20 seconds. Rest for 10 seconds between exercises.

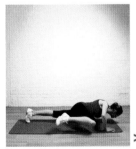

Dragon Push-up (see page 95)

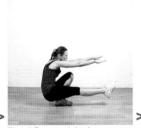

Pistol Squat, right (see page 78)

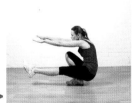

Pistol Squat, left

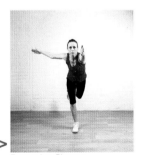

Power Ice Skaters (see page 75)

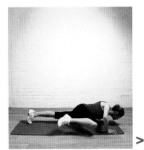

Dragon Push-up

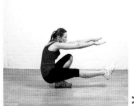

Pistol Squat, right

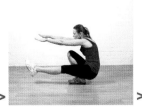

Pistol Squat, left

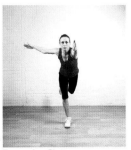

Power Ice Skaters

AMRAP ONE | Complete the following sequence **LOWER BODY AND CORE** | TIME: **5 MINUTES**
of exercises. Complete as many rounds as possible in 5 minutes.

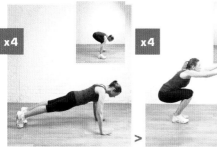 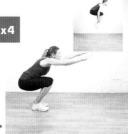 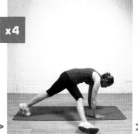 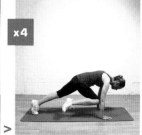

Bear Leap and Reaches (see page 67) > Bear Tucks (see page 84) > Grasshoppers (see page 68–9) > Cross Mountain Climbers (see page 66)

AMRAP TWO | Complete the following sequence **UPPER BODY AND CORE** | TIME: **5 MINUTES**
of exercises. Complete as many rounds as possible in 5 minutes.

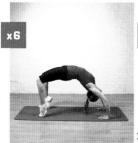 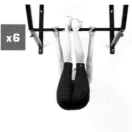 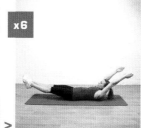 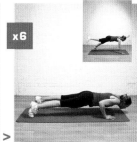

Reverse Push-ups (see page 89) > Toes to Bar (see page 93) > Abdominal Rocks (see page 74) > Tri to Superman Pushes (see page 98)

AMRAP THREE | Complete the following sequence **WHOLE BODY** | TIME: **3 MINUTES**
of exercises. Complete as many rounds as possible in 3 minutes.

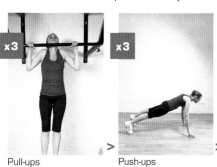 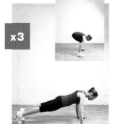 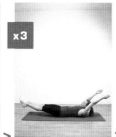 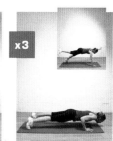

Pull-ups (see page 90) > Push-ups (see page 94) > Bear Leaps and Reaches (see page 67) > Abdominal Rocks (see page 74) > Tri to Superman to Pushes (see page 98)

BODYWEIGHT DENSITY

DENSITY ONE | LOWER BODY AND ABDOMINALS | TIME: **3 MINUTES**

Complete each of the following exercises for 30 seconds back to back.

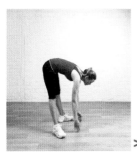

Inchworm (see page 70)

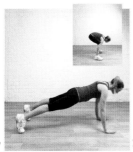

Bear Leap and Reach (see page 67)

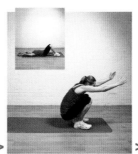

Squat to Abdominal Roll-out to Standing (see page 81)

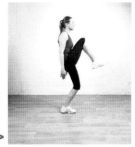

High Knees (see page 76)

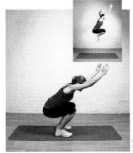

Bear Squats (see page 82)

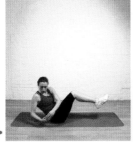

Russian Twist (see page 73)

7 | FUEL AND RECOVERY

'Fuel well. Train regularly.'

If you train with purpose and want to get results, you have to understand that you cannot out-train a bad diet. In other words, if you do all the press-ups in the world but eat trash you won't get a six-pack.

I always hear people saying, 'Great, I've been to the gym so now I can eat burgers and not feel guilty!' But it doesn't work like that.

Yes, afford yourself the occasional treat night out, but don't kid yourself that the gym is a valid excuse to eat badly and still expect great results.

Understand that good nutrition is *the* building block to great fitness and looking good.

It has taken many years for me to understand the importance of a healthy and balanced approach to nutrition. No one taught me in school how to eat for life. I wish they had! Instead, I've had to learn it the hard way – by mistakes, a lot of trial and error and a ton of research and reading!

Despite having above average fitness, when I was younger I never had the toned physique that we all associate with epic fitness. I was strong but I never looked ripped! But I now know that when a good diet, an intense workout regime and a positive mental attitude all come together, you will be in better physical health with a body to be proud of.

It's common sense, of course, but it needs stating clearly: poor food choices that offer little or no nutritional value will always have a negative impact on your training regime. Believe me, I can categorically confirm that a true six-pack is made as much in the kitchen as it is during your workouts.

So put the same energy, discipline and focus into eating right and the results will follow. I promise you.

> " The good news is that rest and
> recovery are fundamental to
> achieving your fitness goals.
> Enjoy – you've earned it! "

A NATURAL AND REAL APPROACH

The basic principles of my natural and real approach to nutrition revolve around eating foods that are as close to their natural and complete state as possible, free from additives or preservatives, and with as few artificial ingredients as you can manage. Go for the best-quality foods available, organic where possible.

People say: 'Oh, that will cost so much more.' But the truth is that if you shop smart and make a lot of your own dishes you needn't spend a fortune to eat right. Beer and ready-made meals aren't always the cheap option – in more ways than one.

I aim to live by these simple, natural eating rules to stay strong, lean and healthy.

Eat:

- grass-fed meats
- organic fish/seafood
- organic fresh fruits and vegetables
- organic free-range eggs
- organic nuts and seeds
- organic healthy oils (olive, walnut, flaxseed, macadamia, avocado, coconut)

Limit:

- potatoes
- dairy
- refined sugar
- processed foods
- carbs such as bread, pasta and rice
- table salt
- refined vegetable oils
- alcohol

FUEL FOR LIVING

'Train hard, eat clean, rest well and be consistent – and watch the athlete inside you emerge.'

The fuel for living concept can be traced back to our forefathers, those hunter-gathers who ate only what they could find and therefore what they were naturally meant to eat. In today's modern, convenience-focused world, we choose to develop and eat foods that satisfy our tastebuds rather than nutrient-rich foods that will fuel our bodies and help them perform better in our day-to-day activities.

A critical step in my personal health and fitness journey was to re-address my relationship with nutrition. I needed to start thinking of what I ate as fuel for living and take responsibility for my body's reaction to the choice of food that was making up my diet.

The biggest changes I made were to portion sizes and percentages of the groups of food I ate. I reduced portion sizes and began to follow a balanced diet made up of 40% carbohydrates (mainly from fruit and veggies), 40% protein (limiting red meat) and 20% good fats.

Although my diet was nutrient-rich, just changing and cleaning it up slightly had a massive impact on my fitness gains and helped reduce body fat. I added way more green vegetables, ate much more white meat than red and increased the frequency with which I ate oily fish to twice a week. I started to really limit refined sugar and simple carbs, like potatoes, breads and pasta, as well as dairy and saturated fats from processed meat like sausages.

The biggest lesson was then learning how to make healthy food taste delicious. Nowadays it's so much easier than it used to be because of the online resources and recipes available to complement this type of healthy eating.

For example, when we want a pizza I make a base from cauliflower – just check it out online!

Or I make chocolate in 2 minutes from coconut oil, raw cacao and natural maple syrup. Both the pizza and the chocolate would blow your mind, they taste so good, I promise!

Healthy eating requires re-educating our tastebuds to wean them off the salt, sugar and fat that hide the great taste of real food, as well as re-educating our minds on how we can make healthy recipes that taste amazing.

Just commit to the learning process and you will get the hang of it, and commit to become a master of researching great healthy, wholefood recipes.

I do two key things: the first is to buy only healthy ingredients. The second is to look up great online recipes that I can cook using only those ingredients. Day by day this means eating healthily is relatively easy, as well as being fun, nutritious and an endeavour that pays dividends towards my fitness goals.

The truth is that to cover nutrition properly requires a whole book and I will write that book some time soon. I want to call it: *Your Life – Fuel for It.* So watch this space! But in the meantime, get started on these solid principles and incorporate them into your life and training, and you will see a huge difference.

In short: good nutrition is critical to great fitness. Embrace that fact.

For 80% of the time I choose to eat a diet that is rich in good-quality fresh fruits, vegetables, good fats, proteins and complex carbohydrates. I am not a qualified specialist in nutrition, but I have tried and tested bad diets and I have learnt, found and researched what really works; and I can confirm that when I eat a diet rich in simple carbohydrates, excess sugars and bad fats my body struggles to break down the food. As a result my workouts suffer, lethargy kicks in and I have to look harder to find that elusive six-pack.

By no means am I telling you to eat a natural and real approach for ever and ever

FOOD GROUPS

Carbohydrates

Our bodies use carbohydrates for energy and there are two types:

Simple carbohydrates (sugar): high in refined sugars and can disrupt your energy levels. For example: white breads, white rice, white pasta, cakes, etc.

Complex carbohydrates (starches): high in sugars but release energy more slowly and stabilize your energy levels. For example: wholewheat pasta, brown rice, rye bread, quinoa, etc.

These complex carbs are way healthier but I personally limit (but don't exclude) these from my diet.

Protein

Protein helps our bodies grow and build muscle. Proteins/essential amino acids are an energy source that helps us burn calories and promotes weight loss.

Fats

Our bodies need good fats to grow and to process vitamins. These fats provide energy for longer bursts of energy.

amen. You and I are human, and life would be pretty restrictive and boring if we lived by the book all the time! That's why I work on an 80:20 ratio. I eat as natural and as lean as I can for 80% of the time and then enjoy the occasional treat and meal out for the rest of the time. Everything in moderation.

FUEL FOR EXERCISE

Your energy levels throughout the day will be determined by your pre- and post-training fuel. It has taken me a whole lot of workouts to get this right! This is trial and error, so use your progress diaries to track and monitor what does and doesn't work for you (see Appendix, page 203).

Pre-workout

I find eating before a workout is essential – it helps fuel my workout and maintain energy levels at high intensities throughout.

The majority of my training is done in the morning, so I treat my breakfast as my pre-workout meal and aim to eat it one hour before I train. One of the best ways to start the day is with a green smoothie.

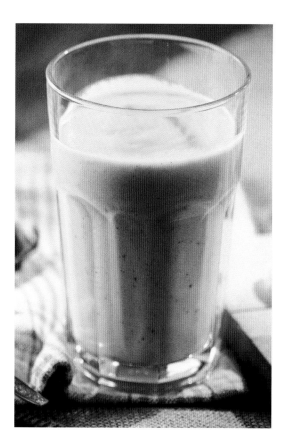

Bear's Kick-start Smoothie

- a banana
- a handful of raw oats
- a handful organic raw kale or organic raw spinach
- a whole organic cucumber (with the skin on it and blended)
- 1 tsp clean greens powder (mine contains spirulina, wheatgrass, kale and sprouts)
- iced water
- fresh ginger, peeled and chopped, to taste

Pop everything together in a blender and blitz! (By the way, juicers just strip all the skin and fibre out of fruit and veg, so I always blend instead.)

As an alternative to my kick-start green smoothie, try a mix of these as a healthy, nutrient-rich breakfast.

- non-whey protein powder with almond milk and a banana, some berries and honey blended with some ice and a handful of oats
- free-range scrambled eggs, the ultimate fast food (and the yolks are great)
- oats cooked in almond milk
- almond butter and banana on toasted rye bread (delicious!)
- smoked salmon and poached eggs with some rocket, asparagus or other fresh greens

TIP! My preference is for non-whey-based (dairy-free) protein. Hemp, pea and brown rice protein powders are all a great source of protein.

Need something on the run? Make these oat-based pancakes and leave them in the fridge for the morning. I love them topped with maple syrup or almond butter and bananas.

Proteins play a vital role in the recovery process after a hard training session. Add protein to your post-workout meal to assist in the repair and synthesis of muscle.

Oat-based Pancakes

- 4 eggs
- 200g authentic Greek yoghurt (although limit this if you decide to drop dairy, as I have)
- 100g organic oats
- cinnamon, to taste
- ½ teaspoon coconut oil

Break the eggs into a blender, then add the yoghurt, oats and cinnamon. Blend everything together into a thick batter.

Heat the coconut oil in a pan, pour in the batter and cook the pancake until golden, carefully flipping it over when the underside is done.

I always use coconut oil to cook with rather than olive or vegetable oil. It is way healthier and has so many great benefits that get lost in other oils when they are heated. (And you don't taste the coconut flavour, by the way.)

Post-workout

Immediately after my workout I refuel with a protein snack, such as unsalted raw nuts and berries, or apple slices with almond butter, followed by a nutrient-rich protein and carbohydrate meal 1 or 2 hours later.

A few of my essential post-workout meals are:

- grilled grass-fed lean steak with organic greens and sweet potatoes
- organic steamed fish with grilled tomatoes, greens and quinoa
- greens stir-fried with eggs and cashew nuts
- oven-baked grass-fed chicken or turkey with lemon and fresh herbs on a bed of colourful vegetables
- protein powder with almond milk and a banana, some berries and some honey blended with some ice (this smoothie is a great, simple, go-to source of healthy protein and nutrients)

NEED A HEALTHY DESSERT?

I am a sucker for a good dessert – to me a main meal feels incomplete without one, but we are all different. My staple choices are either a few squares of home-made dark chocolate; tapioca made with almond milk, a bit of honey, smashed banana, protein powder and honey; or a killer sticky toffee date pudding made with no dairy, white sugar or white flour! (I substitute coconut oil for butter, stevia for sugar and almond flour for white flour – and it tastes amazing!) Again, you don't need a huge bowlful to get the satisfaction of a good pudding. That's the key with desserts.

SUPPLEMENTS

I am very wary of a lot of synthetic supplements and the limit mine to the following:

- Juice Plus+®, which is a natural source of raw fruit and veggies
- a good omega 3-6-9 capsule
- some pro-biotic powder
- a vitamin D3 supplement

Beyond that I aim for all my goodness to come from good, healthy, life-giving, wholefood sources.

A quick and simple guide to check how well hydrated you are is to check the colour of your urine. Put simply: the better hydrated you are, the lighter the colour of your pee will be. Don't let yourself get dehydrated. Your muscles and body need the fluids. And keep away from sugar-laden rehydration drinks. Get the minerals and salts naturally! (I love coconut water to help with this.)

As I've mentioned, optimum hydration levels during your workout will keep you energized for longer and make your workouts more effective. This means drinking plenty of fluids before, during and after your workout. I aim for 500ml still water 45 minutes prior to a workout. Whilst I am working out, I sip water little and often during rest intervals to help replace any fluid I lose through sweat to maintain the intensity of my workout.

Your post-workout fluid requirement depends on how intensely you've worked out. On top of the recommended 2 litres a day, I replace any water I've lost during my session and use the 'pee colour' indicator to measure my level of hydration periodically throughout the day. Oh, and don't drink your pee unless your life is on the line and you are really well hydrated beforehand!

Staying Hydrated

Yep, I'm going to talk about pee, which you know is a subject close to my heart! Staying hydrated is really important for keeping your energy levels up, helping your body metabolize food and also enabling you to maximize the benefits of your workout.

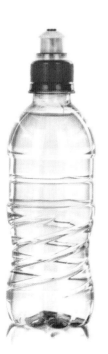

1. HYDRATED

2. HYDRATED

3. HYDRATED

4. DEHYDRATED

5. DEHYDRATED

6. DEHYDRATED

7. SEVERELY DEHYDRATED

8. SEVERELY DEHYDRATED

> Keep your workouts short, dynamic and fun – and they will soon become a life-long positive habit.

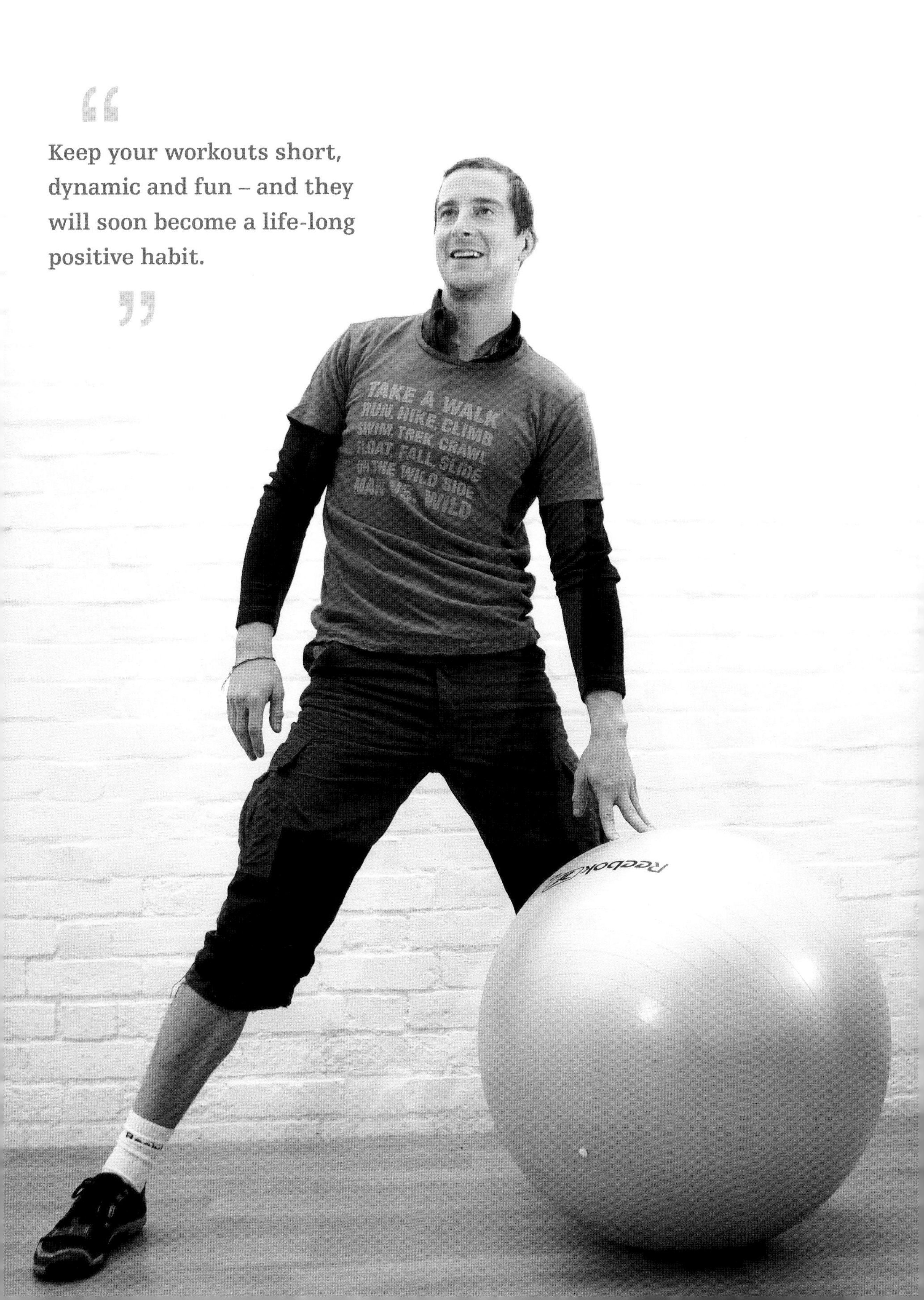

TRACKING YOUR PROGRESS

'Believe in yourself and concentrate on how far you have come on your fitness journey, not how far you have to go.'

PHYSICAL ACTIVITY READINESS QUESTIONNAIRE (PARQ)

Regular physical activity is great fun and the health benefits are tremendous! Being more active is very safe for most of you guys, but some of you may wish to check with your doctor before you get stuck into the workouts and become physically more active.

If you are new to fitness and exercising, we advise you start by answering the questions below.

If you are aged between 15 and 69, this PARQ will tell you if you should check with your doctor before you start.

If you are aged over 69 and you are not used to being very active, we advise you to check with your doctor before trying the workouts, especially the Hero ones!

Common sense is your best guide when you answer these questions. Read the questions carefully and answer each one honestly.

Remember: it's your life – train for it.

YES	NO	
		1. Has your doctor ever said that you have a heart condition and that you should only do physical activity recommended by a doctor?
		2. Do you feel pain in your chest when you do physical activity?
		3. In the past month, have you had chest pain when you were not doing physical activity?
		4. Has a doctor ever told you that you have asthma?
		5. Has a doctor ever told you that you have diabetes?
		6. Do you lose your balance because of dizziness or do you lose consciousness?
		7. Do you have a bone or a joint problem that could be made worse by a change in your physical activity?
		8. Is your doctor currently prescribing drugs (for example, water pills) for your blood pressure or heart condition?
		9. Do you know of ANY other reason why you should not do physical activity?

If you answered YES to one or more questions:

We advise you talk with your doctor by phone or in person before you embark on the workouts and BEFORE you complete the fitness evaluation. Inform your doctor about the PARQ and highlight which questions you answered YES.

■ You may be able to do any activity you want as long as you start slowly and build up gradually. Or you may need to restrict your activities to those that are safe for you. Discuss with your doctor the different kinds of workouts you wish to take part in and follow his/her advice.

■ If you are not ready for these workouts just yet but do wish to start exercising for fitness, you may wish to find out which community programmes are safe and helpful for you in your local area.

If you answered NO to all questions:

If you answered NO honestly to all PARQ questions, you can be reasonably sure that you can:

- Start becoming much more physically active – if it is new, begin slowly and build up gradually. This is the safest and easiest way to go.

- Complete the fitness test (see page 202). This is an excellent way to determine your basic fitness so that you can plan the best way for you to start your fitness journey.

When to delay becoming much more active:

- If you are not feeling well because of a temporary illness such as a cold or a fever – wait till you feel better.

- If you are or may be pregnant – talk to your doctor before you start becoming more active.

> If your health changes so that you answer YES to any of the questions on the previous page, tell your fitness or health professional and ask whether you should change your workout plan.

MAPPING YOUR BODY

Your starting point is to document, track and assess your fitness levels before you embark on your new training regime. I appreciate that if, like me, you are not a natural athlete it can be a little bit daunting, but don't feel negative about your starting point or fear that your journey may be a long one. The important thing to remember is that beginning is always the hardest thing – and if you're reading this, you have already started your journey.

By creating a starting point and tracking your progress you will be able to see how quickly you progress. Now grab a camera, pencil and tape measure and let's get started.

Taking pictures, making memories

A great way to measure your progress is to use photographs. Before and after pictures are a great way of visibly tracking both the subtle and the dramatic body changes in your fitness journey. (Having to take my shirt off regularly on TV is great motivation to keep fit, and I can see from the TV shows over the years when I was doing well and less well on that front!)

Take full-length pictures. Make sure you can see your body. Ask someone to take pictures of your front, back and side profile. You can use the Training and Progress Diary (see page 203) to make a note of the day of the week, the time of day and how you feel after you have taken these pictures.

> Remember, you don't have to share your before and after pictures with social media! Keep it private is my advice. The pictures are to track your own personal progress. But if you do want to share your experiences and your fitness progress (and it can be good motivation, although not always easy viewing!) use #yourlifetrainforit to get involved.

Once you've successfully completed six weeks of your new training routine, take a second set of pictures in the same positions and poses as the first set. Try to wear the same clothes and take the pictures at the same time of day as your original pictures. Continue to take progress pictures every six weeks until you reach your fitness goals.

Measure your body

This is one of the most effective and important tools to use in tracking your fitness progress. Weigh yourself if you must and record it, but be aware that in isolation measuring your weight is not the most accurate indicator of progress – as you build lean muscle, you may in fact put on weight. Standing on the scales will give you an idea of overall weight loss, but not of body-fat reduction.

You can achieve more accurate measurement of your progress by using a tape measure to check different parts of the body that will be used to map out body-shape changes. Here are a few handy tips for making sure you get accurate results each time you measure:

- Stick to the same time of day and use the same tape measure each time you record your measurements.
- Make sure you take your measurements in the same places each time. Try to use body markers as a guide – for example freckles, moles or scars.
- Don't hold your breath or suck your tummy in – be honest!
- Record your measurements for the following areas:

  - **Neck** – measure around your neck's mid-point.
  - **Shoulders** – stand up straight and measure the circumference around both shoulders.

  - **Chest** – wrap the tape measure around your chest and measure in line with your nipples.
  - **Bicep** – take two measurements. Find the mid-point on your upper arm and measure round with and without tensing the bicep muscle.
  - **High waist** – find your bottom rib and measure around your torso.
  - **Waist** – place your finger in your belly button and wrap the tape measure around, in line with your belly button. Make sure the tape measure is straight all the way around.
  - **Hips** – locate the widest part of your hips and measure right round.
  - **Thigh** – measure round at the mid-point between your knee and the top of your leg.
  - **Calf** – measure round at the mid-point of your lower leg.

THE FITNESS TEST

OK, you have mapped out your body measurements. Now it's time to evaluate your physical fitness. The most effective way to do this is with a fitness test.

This test is individual to you and the only person you need to compare yourself to is you, over a six-week period. You should perform the fitness test every six weeks until you reach your desired fitness goal. The sole purpose of this fitness test is for self-evaluation and to measure the positive steps in your self-improvement.

Right, let's get our fitness gear on, warm up and get started!

How to complete the fitness test

Before you get started, make sure you do the following:

- Learn the moves before you embark on the test (see Exercise Library, pages 24–127).
- Make a note of your scores using the Training and Progress Diary (see pages 203–6).
- Take the test at the same time of day every six weeks.

The test

1. Warm up first (see Bodyweight Warm-up, pages 132–3).

2. Complete each of the following exercises for 1 minute, resting for 30 seconds in between exercises. Record your results in the space provided.

EXERCISE	BEGINNER	INTERMEDIATE	ADVANCED	No OF REPS
Push-ups	Knees down	On toes	Power	
Russian Twists	Feet down	Feet up	3-point Russian Twist	
Burpees	No jump	With jump	With a tuck jump	
Goblet Squat to Military Overhead Press	Light weight 8kg	Medium weight 12kg	Heavy weight 16kg	
100 Double-hand Kettlebell Swings	8kg	12kg	16kg	
Plank	Basic	Single leg	Single-arm Kettlebell	

3. Perform a plank and measure how long you can hold the Low Plank position for.

If you exceed 2 minutes, advance to a Single-leg Plank.
If you exceed 2 minutes for a Single-leg Plank, progress to a Single-arm Kettlebell Plank.
Rest for 1 minute.

4. Flexibility test:

- Sit with your back against a wall and your legs out straight in front.
- Hinge at your hips and fold forward at the hips – take care not to round your back as you reach your hands forward.
- Continue to fold with a flat back as far as you can.
- Make a note of how far you were able to reach – for example to your shins, past your ankles, toes or beyond. Ask a partner or friend to take a photo for your records.

5. Rest, recover and complete a whole-body cool-down (see pages 138–9).

TWELVE-WEEK TRAINING AND PROGRESS DIARY

'Stop competing with others and start competing with yourself.'

Date: _____

What is your motivation to start? _____
_____
_____
_____

Your ultimate fitness goal: _____
_____
_____
_____

Short-term fitness goals:

■ 3 weeks _____
_____

■ 6 weeks _____

Medium-term fitness goals:

■ 12 weeks _____
_____

■ 18 weeks _____
_____

Long-term fitness goals:

■ 4 months _____
_____

■ 8 months _____
_____

■ 12 months _____
_____

WEEK ONE   Body Mapping

Date: _____   Time: _____

Pictures:

front	side	back

Weight: _____

Measurements: _____

Focus areas for muscle definition:
_____

_____

Focus areas for body-fat reduction:
_____

_____

Neck

Shoulders

Chest

Bicep

High Waist

Waist

Hips

Thigh

Calf

Physical Mapping

Complete your fitness evaluation and record your results on the chart below.

EXERCISE	BEGINNER	INTERMEDIATE	ADVANCED	No OF REPS	
Push-ups	Knees down	On toes	Power		
Russian Twists	Feet down	Feet up	3-point Russian Twist		
Burpees	No jump	With jump	With a tuck jump		
Goblet Squat to Military Overhead Press	Light weight 8kg	Medium weight 12kg	Heavy weight 16kg		
100 Double-hand Kettlebell Swings	8kg	12kg	16kg		
Plank	Basic	Single leg	Single-arm Kettlebell		

How do you feel?

Strong ☐   Weak ☐   Energized ☐   Motivated ☐   Focused ☐   Challenged ☐

WEEK SIX Body Mapping

Date: _____   Time: _____

Pictures:

front	side	back

Weight: _____

Measurements: _____

Focus areas for muscle definition:
_____

_____

Focus areas for body-fat reduction:
_____

_____

Neck

Shoulders

Chest

Bicep

High Waist

Waist

Hips

Thigh

Calf

Physical Mapping

Complete your fitness evaluation and record your results on the chart below.

EXERCISE	BEGINNER	INTERMEDIATE	ADVANCED		No OF REPS
Push-ups	Knees down	On toes	Power		
Russian Twists	Feet down	Feet up	3-point Russian Twist		
Burpees	No jump	With jump	With a tuck jump		
Goblet Squat to Military Overhead Press	Light weight 8kg	Medium weight 12kg	Heavy weight 16kg		
100 Double-hand Kettlebell Swings	8kg	12kg	16kg		
Plank	Basic	Single leg	Single-arm Kettlebell		

How do you feel?

Strong ☐   Weak ☐   Energized ☐   Motivated ☐   Focused ☐   Challenged ☐

WEEK TWELVE   Body Mapping

Date: _____   Time: _____

Pictures:

front	**side**	**back**

Weight: _____

Measurements: _____

Focus areas for muscle definition: _____

_____

Focus areas for body-fat reduction: _____

_____

Neck

Shoulders

Chest

Bicep

High Waist

Waist

Hips

Thigh

Calf

Physical Mapping

Complete your fitness evaluation and record your results on the chart below.

EXERCISE	BEGINNER	INTERMEDIATE	ADVANCED	No OF REPS
Push-ups	Knees down	On toes	Power	
Russian Twists	Feet down	Feet up	3-point Russian Twist	
Burpees	No jump	With jump	With a tuck jump	
Goblet Squat to Military Overhead Press	Light weight 8kg	Medium weight 12kg	Heavy weight 16kg	
100 Double-hand Kettlebell Swings	8kg	12kg	16kg	
Plank	Basic	Single leg	Single-arm Kettlebell	

How do you feel?

Strong ☐   Weak ☐   Energized ☐   Motivated ☐   Focused ☐   Challenged ☐

FINAL WORD

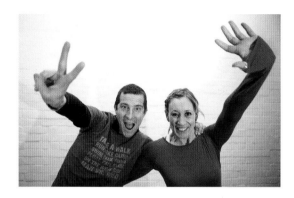

Remember, everything you have read here is meaningless unless you act on it. Knowledge without action has no power. You have to go through the rain to reach the rainbow; you have to sacrifice some time and energy to get the results you want.

This programme will make that journey to a fitter, stronger and healthier you as fun, effective and short as I believe is possible, but still you have to do it!

So be disciplined with yourself. Self-discipline is such a life-enhancing character trait to develop. Be committed – remember, commitment is doing the thing you said you would do long after the mood you said it in has left you!

Be consistent. Be determined. Good, worthwhile things in life never come easy.

But also enjoy regular treats and down weekends, reward yourself, relish the journey. It shouldn't all be ball-busting and we all need a break occasionally!

Final thing is to try to find a buddy to do this programme with. It makes it so much easier to achieve great results when you have a training partner. I know this from SAS Selection; having a best buddy to train with and share the highs and lows made a critical difference to me.

So there we go, do all this and the dynamic survivor, the powerful athlete and the lean you will emerge – and I can't wait to hear your story. Write and tell me, send me your pictures! I love hearing about your journeys. Such stories remind me that we are all in this together.

Just like you, I am on the same road – a road without a final destination, but a road where the journey itself is the mission.

It is all about being fitter, healthier and stronger, day by day, so we are best equipped to embrace the great adventure called life.

'So, keep on going – don't quit! It's your life. Train for it.'

Natalie's Acknowledgements

Thank you to my husband, Mike; sisters Kirstie and Jodie; and to my beautiful daughter, Amelie. You have all had to be patient so often and your love and support know no bounds. Huge thanks to my mum and dad; you have never stopped supporting me and always said my personality and enthusiasm would inspire people. I hope that this book inspires many.

A big shout out to our editor, Rebecca Wright; it has been a joy working with you. And many thanks to Bobby Birchall for his ability to bring the design vision to life.

Finally, my sincere gratitude goes to Bear. Your constant inspiration, determination, effort and belief have made this an incredible experience that I will remember for the rest of my life. You have helped me grow and flourish, and I will always be grateful. I can't wait to continue on the next stage of the journey with you.

TRANSWORLD PUBLISHERS
61–63 Uxbridge Road, London W5 5SA
A Random House Group Company
www.transworldbooks.co.uk

First published in Great Britain
in 2014 by Bantam Press
an imprint of Transworld Publishers

Copyright © Bear Grylls Ventures and Natalie Summers 2014

Photography by Jeremy Prout except pages 2, 5, 6, 7, 9, 27, 29 (top right), 35 (background), 47, 54, 58–9, 62–3 (background), 68–9 (background), 71 (background), 79, 83, 88, 91, 97, 101, 117, 123, 127, 129, 140, 143, 151, 159, 166, 171, 191, 197, 207 courtesy of BGV, and pages 194, 196, 204–6 © Shutterstock.

Bear Grylls has asserted his right under the Copyright,
Designs and Patents Act 1988 to be identified as the author of this work.

A CIP catalogue record for this book
is available from the British Library.

ISBN 9780593074190

The health and fitness information in this book has been compiled by way of general guidance in relation to the specific subjects addressed. It is not intended as a substitute for medical advice. Please consult your GP or healthcare professional before performing the exercises described in this book, particularly if you are pregnant, elderly or have chronic or recurring medical conditions. Do not attempt any of the exercises while under the influence of alcohol or drugs. Discontinue any exercise that causes you pain or severe discomfort and consult a medical expert. So far as the author is aware the information given is correct and up to date as at the time of publication. The author and publishers disclaim, as far as the law allows, any liability arising directly or indirectly from the use, or misuse, of the information contained in this book.

Addresses for Random House Group Ltd companies outside the UK
can be found at: www.randomhouse.co.uk
The Random House Group Ltd Reg. No. 954009

The Random House Group Limited supports the Forest Stewardship Council® (FSC®), the leading international forest-certification organisation. Our books carrying the FSC label are printed on FSC®-certified paper. FSC is the only forest-certification scheme supported by the leading environmental organisations, including Greenpeace. Our paper procurement policy can be found at
www.randomhouse.co.uk/environment

Designed by Bobby&Co
Typeset in Eurostyle and Egyptienne
Printed and bound in Germany by
Mohn Media Mohndruck GmbH

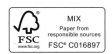